Managing Your Doctor

HOW TO GET
THE BEST POSSIBLE
HEALTH CARE

DR. ARTHUR S. FREESE

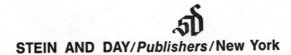

STEIN AND DAY/*Publishers*/New York

First published by Stein and Day, Incorporated, in 1975
Copyright © 1974 by Arthur S. Freese
Library of Congress Catalog No. 74-78534
All rights reserved
Designed by David Miller
Printed in the United States of America
Stein and Day/Publishers/Scarborough House,
Briarcliff Manor, N.Y. 10510
ISBN 0-8128-1728-1

To Dr. Joseph L. Bell, in deepest appreciation for generous help and insightful advice that provided much depth and direction.

Contents

Why You Should Learn Doctor-Management   9

PART I
*What You Must Know to Protect
Yourself in Dealing with Doctors,
Hospitals, Dentists, and Medical
Emergencies*

1 Whom Should You Seek as a Family Doctor?   19
2 How to Find and Check a Family Doctor   26
3 Finding and Using the Right Hospital   36
4 Surgery Can Be Murder: How to Protect Yourself   47
5 How to Get Life-Saving Help in Medical Emergencies   57
6 What You Must Know to Find the Right Psychiatrist   70
7 How to Find and Use a Dentist—without Being Used   80

PART II
*Special Problems in Managing Your
Doctors: How to Keep Yourself Safe
from Medical Mayhem*

8 Protecting Yourself against X-rays   95
9 The Medical Drug Scene, the Doctor, and You   105

10 Guarding against the Miracle Drugs
    that Spell "Murder"   120
11 Managing the Medical Drug-Pushers:
    Physician, Heal Thyself!   130
12 Painkillers, Placebos, and Physicians   141

PART III
*Doctor Talk and What It Really
Means to You*

13 What Your Doctor Must Be Made to Say
    —and What You Should Never Omit   153
14 Is There a Doctor in the House—for the Gay
    People, the Women, the Elderly, the Teenagers?   165
15 How to Get Help for Your Sexual Problems   175
16 Your Home Medical Library:
    Books that Will Help You to Manage Your Doctor   184

Bibliography   189

Why You Should Learn Doctor-Management

Today's medical care is a mixture of professional brilliance and greedy bungling; of near-genius surgical procedures and totally unnecessary ones; of lives daringly saved and others needlessly wasted. Between these extremes of our health-care world are countless gradations through which you must learn to thread your way in order to safeguard your own health.

Modern medicine is truly a matter of triumph and tragedy: a woman in her mid-sixties was admitted to an East Coast hospital for routine thyroid-gland surgery. Just as the operation was successfully completed and the wound was being sutured, the anesthesia machine produced an explosion whose full force struck the woman; she died four and a half hours later.... A man received x-ray treatments for the eczema on his legs from a non-specialist doctor; excessive radiation produced third-degree burns, and both legs had to be amputated.... Experts estimate that several million unnecessary operations are performed annually, resulting in tens of thousands of avoidable deaths.

But an Indianapolis schoolteacher has become the first man to live with a transplanted heart for more than five years, and the oldest transplanted kidney has now been functioning for some fifteen years. A forty-nine-year-old New England woman recently became the first person to survive open-heart surgery, kidney removal, and a kidney transplant.

Still, hundreds of thousands of sufferers can get no relief from physical pain, while others become addicted to medications mistakenly prescribed for emotional distress. And by a conservative estimate, every year 1.5 million people require hospitalization for adverse reactions to medication. A recent study has revealed that almost two-thirds of the patients getting antibiotics in seven community hospitals showed no evidence of any infection (so why these drugs?)—and the miracle drugs are known to cause a high proportion of adverse reactions.

Yet, since World War II, powerful new medications have revolutionized medicine, giving man control over many infections and diseases for the first time in history. Meanwhile, a tiny electronic device keeps the heart of Supreme Court Justice William O. Douglas beating seventy times a minute, day in and day out; and a 105-year-old woman has just had the batteries in her pacemaker recharged. For the first time it is possible to talk of cures for a number of cancers—Hodgkin's disease, at least one form of leukemia (acute lymphocytic), cancer of the lymph tissues, and seven others.

Why Is Doctor-Management Important for You?

The answer is clear if we only look at the figures. Every month, 750 out of 1,000 Americans suffer some ailment; 250 seek a physician's help, and about 100 are hospitalized. Americans consult doctors an average of 4.5 times per year. What are the chances that these patients—that you as a health-care "consumer"—will get the correct treatment?

The chances are slim, to judge by the anger and frustration Americans in general feel about the health care they receive and the doctors who provide it. The broad-based and knowledgeable Citizens Board of Inquiry into Health Services (recently formed, with half its members either physicians or leaders in the health-care field) has studied the medical consumer in every part of the United States. In their report, *Heal Yourself,* the board says: "Unless one has faced a room of angry consumers . . . one cannot realize the extent or depth of that anger and frustration. . . . Let there be no mistake. The anger is well founded. The deficiencies are real."

A recent Louis Harris poll found that a majority of Americans consider good health even more important than a good job. The purpose of this book is to show how *you* can control the system of fee-for-service care that dominates American medicine today; how *you* can manage your doctor in order to become one of the few who obtain adequate health care; how *you* can bridge the enormous gap between the possible and the available. To do all this, health-care consumers must first exorcize some old misconceptions about their physicians.

The Myth of the Family Doctor

The American public seems to have a fixed notion of the good old-fashioned family doctor of the past—the "Doc" of the TV show *Gunsmoke,* the wise, fatherly practitioner who gave so generously of himself, who was available at any hour of any day, who accepted whatever remuneration his patients could afford—and, most important, who treated the whole person and not just the body part he specialized in.

Sir Luke Fildes portrayed this romanticized figure in his 1891 painting, which still hangs in London's Tate Gallery—the devoted professional sitting by the sick child as dawn breaks, the distraught parents looking on. More than a million engravings of this work are said to have hung in the living rooms of the public and the waiting rooms of physicians, not to mention the countless reproductions that have appeared in advertisements in medical and popular journals, and even on an American postage stamp in 1947.

What is the truth about the doctors of the past, who make our current physicians seem so careless? New York University's Professor Eliot Freidson, one of America's leading medical sociologists and long a student of the medical profession, believes that the ideal family practitioner actually existed only for a brief spot in time, some twenty or thirty years perhaps, early in our own century. Probably only during the Great Depression of the 1930s was there a prototypal family doctor who managed all of a person's medical problems and those of his family, knew parents and children and often grandchildren as well.

As Dr. Freidson has pointed out, the history of medicine is actually only the history of medical discoveries, of the "urban academic medicine which in fact had hardly anything to do with

90 per cent of the population." "Doc" of *Gunsmoke*—if he ever in reality existed--probably wasn't even a physician with a bona fide degree but got what degree he had by mail, if he had one at all. Patent medicines were widely used in the nineteenth century, and self-treatment was more common than professional treatment. Most people actually avoided trained doctors because their only cures—bleeding and purging—were so unpleasant. Not until our own century did medicine become the profession we know today, with licensing and careful controls.

Only after World War I could any patient expect a better than fifty-fifty chance of getting help from a medical practitioner. But the medical practice in this century has seen more revolution than evolution. It has changed so rapidly that most patients have found themselves helplessly seeking a doctor to take charge of all their health needs and act as their medical advocate when dealing with specialists and hospitals.

Who Cares for the Whole Patient?

The problem of medical specialization is hardly a new one, for the ancient Greek historian Herodotus complained of the Egyptian doctors four thousand years ago: "Every physician is for one disease . . . for there are physicians of the eyes, others of the head . . . of the teeth . . . of the belly, others of obscure diseases."

Specialization disappeared with the ancient Egyptians, only to reappear on the medical scene in the nineteenth century. At first specialists were opposed bitterly by general practitioners (G.P.s), called quacks, and even refused admittance into medical societies. By the turn of the century specialists were accepted into the medical family, and the first modern specialty organization appeared during World War I—the American Board of Ophthalmology. Specialists are called "board-certified," and you can see a diploma to this effect on their walls.

Specialization has now come full circle. The American Board of Family Practice certifies a family practitioner (F.P.) as a full specialist if he has received the necessary training—a sort of space age G.P. The change has been radical: whereas, in 1931, 84 per cent of doctors in private practice were G.P.s, this dropped to 45 per cent in 1960 and to 37 per cent in 1965. As of 1972, the American Medical Association (AMA) figures show that only 15.5 per cent of the nation's 357,000 physicians are in general practice. The current revival of family practice will be discussed more fully in the next chapter.

Why You Must Be Your Own Health Manager

When there were few specialists it was simple to get health care—all you had to do was select a G.P. you liked. With the limited medical knowledge and techniques of those times you couldn't go too far wrong, because the doctor didn't have much more than aspirin to work with anyhow. Today the few G.P.s (or F.P.s) around are overburdened and difficult to reach. In short, it's a whole new ball game.

Before World War II a physician could be reasonably certain that the medical knowledge and skills he acquired in training would—with some reading and perhaps an occasional post-graduate course—keep his practice up to date throughout his professional life. But the scientific explosion that came at the time of World War II blasted medicine right out of its comfortable rut; the science of medicine has revolutionized the practice of medicine and kept it whirling like a dervish ever since. Only continuing education—reading helps marginally at best—enables a doctor to keep his practice current.

You Are on Your Own!

That license to practice medicine that you see on your doctor's wall is actually meaningless. It's issued by a state board of examiners and presumably means the practitioner had at least the minimal qualifications for his profession—at the time it was granted. Once given, the certificate is valid for a lifetime unless the doctor is convicted of a crime or gross misbehavior. His license is renewable simply by filling out a questionnaire and paying a fee, and some states do not even require that much. In only fifteen states can a medical license be challenged for professional incompetence.

In January 1973 the Commission on Medical Malpractice (appointed by the United States Secretary of Health, Education, and Welfare) reported an analysis of 342 disciplinary actions taken by state boards—only 12 cases were for professional incompetence. The figure is not surprising, since some states' medical practice acts have not been changed since they were first passed a century or more ago.

What You Can (and Should) Expect from Your Doctor

Today's doctor is a long way from that ideal figure of yester-year: warm, wise, personally committed to his patients. But if you learn to manage the new professional you can get medical care that is better scientifically and technically than ever before.

To get the many benefits the medical profession can provide, you have a right to expect certain things, although you'll have to give up a good many others. First, you should expect and demand top medical know-how in your doctor (we'll discuss the ways you can check this in later chapters) and in any specialist or hospital he sends you to. But don't expect a leisurely discussion—any doctor worth seeing today is sure to be a busy man or woman. Don't expect him or her to listen to a long description of the soreness that dragged on after you played your first tennis of the season.

You do have every right to spend the time necessary for a full discussion of your medical history, your problems and com-plaints—and you should stand on this right or just leave and find another physician. For instance, when Wally mentioned to his new internist that he'd had the mumps (it happened in his thirties), the doctor cut him off with an impatient "Not important" and con-tinued his hurried questioning, only to be interrupted by a tele-phone call. When this was over, Wally insistently went on, "As I was saying, I had the mumps some twenty years ago, and you will find a badly shrunken testicle in your examination." Nevertheless, the physician was surprised to find this condition some minutes later when he examined Wally, who again had to repeat the in-formation. Wisely, Wally never went back to that doctor.

Know what is important in your medical history and current physical condition, and demand that the physician pay attention to these matters. If he doesn't, it's time to start looking for another practitioner (we'll discuss how to find one later in our book). Don't bother a doctor with irrelevant or unimportant details (how sunburns bother you, what your grandmother suffered, or whatever)—otherwise he'll end up ignoring everything you say and you'll fail to get the help you want.

You have a right to enough time to present all your meaningful complaints, for a careful and unhurried examination, a thorough discussion of your condition, and answers to serious questions: what does your raised blood pressure mean, what drugs are being prescribed for you, what side effects are they likely to have, etc.

Don't discuss your minor personal problems (a fight with your wife or your husband's glances at another woman) unless you are dealing with the relatively rare and new family physician, whom we shall meet later. However, if there is something that deeply bothers you, the doctor should be apprised of this fact—he may not get involved in the emotional problem but will assess its importance to any medical problems. The doctor should either help you with sexual or emotional problems or refer you to someone who can.

You *do* have a right to total medical care from your personal doctor: careful regular screening for all physical problems, diseases, or disorders, and an alertness to any indications that emotional or other help outside his competence may be needed. You also have the right to expect that your doctor will refer you to a specialist when one is needed or when you want to allay concern over some major problem (heart condition, diabetes, etc.).

You also have the right to a simple telephone answer when you ask for one. For example, Janice was confused by the diet her doctor recommended for a diabetic complication. When she phoned him for clarification, he was annoyed and gave her an appointment—then charged her a $25 fee for what a five-minute phone call could have resolved. She had been taken advantage of in a way that is unfortunately common today. On the other hand, don't expect a doctor to spend half an hour on the phone discussing a whole range of problems. For this, go into his office and pay his fee, but demand the time for your problems and any necessary reasonable phone consultations as well.

Certainly your doctor should be available to you in any serious or potentially serious situation: "I've developed a severe ringing in my ears since I started this new medicine" ... "I've gotten this severe chest pain I never had before" ... or whatever.

When you deal with specialists, however, you'll have to accept a lot less personal interest and less time during and after visits (we suggest ways of dealing with this later too). Here a family doctor helps because he can often get answers or give you explanations, coordinate your medical care, and in general act as your advocate in complex medical problems involving a number of specialists, each handling his particular field or organ.

Learning what to expect from your doctor is your first step in managing your doctor. After all, your real aim is to get the best possible medical care at a time when true miracles of medical help are possible. This book can show you how.

PART I

What You Must Know to
Protect Yourself in Dealing with
Doctors, Hospitals, Dentists,
and Medical Emergencies

1

Whom Should You Seek as a Family Doctor?

John has a simple attitude toward medicine: "My doctor knows what he's doing and I never ask questions. I just do what he says." This belief may have been safe in the days of the mythical "good old family doctor," but it certainly isn't wise today—not if you value your life or your health. A close look at the doctors themselves will show why you ultimately have to depend on yourself.

Why You Must Be Wary in Choosing Your Doctor

Narcotics addiction, for example, runs thirty to a hundred times higher among physicians than in the general population, and about one out of every six known drug addicts in the United States, England, Holland, France, and Germany is a doctor. One twenty-year study found that physicians take more tranquilizers, sedatives, and stimulants than non-physicians, and a longer study found doctors more likely to have poor marriages, take drugs, and drink heavily. Suicides and violent deaths also run high among physicians, further proof that emotional problems plague their profession. In one decade, in Arizona and Oregon, some 7.5 per cent of doctors were brought up before the state boards of medical examiners for alcoholism, drug dependence, or mental disorders.

The precise effect of these factors on medical practice is unknown, but the Commission on Medical Malpractice has found that nearly 8 per cent of patients' medical charts show evidence of medical injuries, many preventable. And Dr. James A. Visconti, director of the Drug (medication) Information Center at Ohio State University Hospitals, has revealed that in a single recent year nearly 1.5 million patient-visits to doctors' offices and hospitals were due to drug (medication) reactions. Three-quarters of these reactions were actually predictable, and most could have been prevented without losing the beneficial effects of the drugs concerned. Dr. David C. Lewis, a Harvard Medical School professor, surveyed Boston physicians recently and found two-thirds of them agreeing that doctors prescribe too many sedatives, tranquilizers, and amphetamines. Physicians' mishandling has even aided patients' suicide attempts.

How do the mishaps occur? One story is in the files of a large hospital in a West Coast city. On a Sunday, a forty-two-year-old accountant (we'll call him Henry) had a headache. For a week it worsened, and the following Monday his doctor hospitalized him with a diagnosis of hepatitis; on Wednesday he was told to go home to recover. By then Henry was so confused that he couldn't leave the hospital, and another doctor kept him for tests. On Friday, Henry's wife insisted on calling in a neurologist, who ordered special head x-rays that, on Saturday, revealed a mass in the brain. Emergency surgery found and drained a large abscess. Days of coma were followed by slow recovery, and Henry was in bed for more than two weeks following surgery, with no vision and no memory. After a month and a half in the hospital, Henry finally did go home—knowing only his name, address, and phone number, and with much of his vision gone.

Unusual? Not at all. A few years before this, in New York City, a distraught wife was told on the phone by an internist that he'd made an appointment for her husband to discuss his headache with a psychiatrist—at that very moment the now-delirious husband was being wheeled out to an ambulance. The story was almost the same as Henry's except that his wife doubted the doctor sooner, the neurologist and surgeon came earlier. The post-surgery course was similar too, but vision returned almost fully and there was no memory loss despite the days of coma.

General Medical Practice Today

In a large southern city one G.P. sees some sixty patients a day in his office and also makes some house calls. He packs his patients in so tightly that they don't dare speak to him. He notifies them when he's coming for a house call, and the front door must be left unlocked because it wastes as much as two minutes if he has to ring the bell and wait for someone to answer it. He dashes in, rushes to the bedroom to see the sick patient, scrawls a prescription or barks a few words of instruction, and races away. The husband of one patient with heart trouble timed the whole bit—it took exactly a minute and a half. But he doesn't complain. He's afraid he won't be able to find another doctor willing to make house calls.

A doctor from a western state lectures physicians' conventions across the country on how he's automated his practice. He sees an average of forty-four patients a day and never works in the evening. His consultations would seem to average some five minutes a patient. In his office there are three lights over the door of each examining room: different colors and combinations tell when a patient is in the room, when the patient is ready for the doctor, and, for the nurses, where the doctor is. Seeing sixty or more patients a day is not uncommon among G.P.s—even among those who are not automated for efficiency.

Does Anybody Look over Your Doctor's Shoulder?

Only when doctors evaluate one another will health-care quality-control ever be attained—and the medical profession is fighting hard to prevent it. When you hear about peer review or PSRO (Professional Standards Review Organization), this refers to the proposal that other doctors check on the private practitioner. One G.P., who sees some sixty patients a day, nearly became hysterical when discussing this idea. "Filling out forms just like in the hospital, that's what PSRO is all about. We have to fight these things. I don't want to fill out more than one record just like I've been doing. Everybody in our medical society voted to fight it because we don't want anybody to tell us what to do."

Physicians have good reason to fear such evaluations. One widely quoted study revealed that nearly half the doctors in North Carolina were poor or only little better in their practice of medicine, fewer than a third were reasonably satisfactory, one-fifth were quite good, and one-tenth outstanding. Many of the faults were fundamental, such as inadequate examination and history taking. And this study's findings have been confirmed in other sections of the country. It's not just a local phenomenon.

A recent survey of health care of teamsters' families by the Columbia University School of Public Health in New York revealed that the medical care given seven out of ten patients was "less than optimal" (essentially a failure to diagnose adequately the cause of a problem so that the treatment could be appropriate). The disorders that showed poor care were divided equally among heart disease, respiratory disease, intestinal problems, and a potpourri of other ailments. Heart-attack victims were permitted out of bed or sent home too early, evidence of heart trouble was not investigated, and so on.

In short, it doesn't matter where you live. The quality of medical care is questionable even in such life-threatening disorders as heart disease. Anyone who, like our friend John, depends blindly on a doctor whom he never questions is gambling with his life. But the good medical care practiced in America is among the finest in the world, and this is what you must learn to obtain.

Care *vs.* Cure: Why You Need a Generalist

In general, doctors aren't very interested in health. They're much more interested in illness, for their training and practice are in the cure of disease. To public and physicians alike, health care and medical cure seem one and the same, but they are actually quite different. Cure is meant to combat disease, a particular action to attack a specific illness; but health care (maintenance, if you prefer) is the day-to-day continuous medical effort to keep the individual well and prevent illness. The medical specialist, with rare exceptions (the ophthalmologist with his calls for regular check-ups is one), is interested only in the disorders of his particular bit of your anatomy. He cares and knows little about your over-all health.

This is why you need a generalist, a doctor who will act as the captain of your health team, who will direct the entire orchestra, as it were: the medical man or woman who will accept responsibility for your health on a continuing basis, responding to your illnesses but also advising you of ways to maintain health and minimize sickness. Most of all, the generalist should have the resources and the will to arrange for specialists when needed, to coordinate and explain the total effort in a complex problem or a prolonged chronic one, to support both the sufferer and his family, to answer their questions.

Who Should Your Generalist Be?

The one who automatically springs to mind, of course, is the G.P. of mythical memory, but he's pretty well gone, along with the steam locomotive and the horse-and-buggy—gone simply because G.P.s can't provide the protection and advantages of today's sophisticated techniques.

The young physician interested in general practice today enters a new specialty (it was recognized officially only in 1969), that of family practice. This family practitioner (F.P.) is trained to handle everything the G.P. did but with today's latest scientific expertise. The F.P. is a specialist who has passed his boards—special examinations—in family practice, as the internist has in internal medicine. He has undergone thorough training to protect you in many ways. You can identify the F.P., as you can any other specialist, by the diploma on his wall, which attests to his certification by the American Board of Family Practice. If he's only a member of the Academy of Family Practice he's not a specialist, not truly an F.P., although many G.P.s today like to call themselves family practitioners because it's fashionable.

The board-certified F.P. is trained to handle 70, 80, 90 per cent of your family's health-care and medical needs. In the traditionally specialized areas, this F.P. should be able to care for three-quarters of your neurological problems (such as headaches, stroke, and epilepsy), most skin disorders, most pediatrics, and a great deal of obstetrics (as Dr. Len H. Andrus, a professor of family practice at the University of California, at Davis, pointed out, Holland has a very low maternal death rate, but most Dutch babies are delivered at home by midwives).

There are some forty departments or divisions of family practice in about a third of our medical schools. Many who head these courses hope that the F.P. will even bring back house calls, using a new sophistication and expertise to practice what amounts to environmental medicine. The F.P. who goes into the home would point out health hazards there, such as medicine chests that permit children to get at dangerous drugs (aspirin kills some hundred children every year), slippery bathtubs, or loose rugs that can be serious hazards to the elderly. The F.P. will bring a new concept of continuous health care and preventive medicine to the medical profession in the future.

Unfortunately, the certified F.P. is still hard to find; there were only some 5,800 in the United States as of January 1974. However, almost 2,000 more are taking F.P. residencies (the three-year or more hospital F.P. programs that prepare the young doctor to take his board examinations), and the numbers are growing rapidly. The need for family doctors is clearly being recognized, and more young doctors are attracted to this badly needed specialty.

With so few of these generalist-specialists yet around, you'll probably have to divide your family's health care among the traditional specialties: an internist for the adults (probably a gynecologist as well), a pediatrician, and possibly even a doctor in adolescent medicine for the teenagers (more about this new specialist in Chapter 14). You can check the specialization of internist, gynecologist, or pediatrician by looking for the diploma that shows he is board-certified.

The internist's situation is a little more complicated because he usually practices both general internal medicine (a specialist in general medicine) and his sub-specialty (diabetes, rheumatic disorders, or whatever). To make a living he usually has to provide general health care to a cadre of patients. With his expertise he can offer the best in general medicine to the adult in much the same way as the F.P. and, hopefully, with much the same personal interest and involvement.

Points to Remember

1. Physicians have problems just as everyone else does. You cannot afford to trust a physician blindly just because he has that M.D. degree and license to practice tacked up on his wall. In fact, you should examine his diplomas carefully to see if he has board certification and in what specialty.

2. A generalist (an internist or an F.P.), someone to direct the orchestration of your medical care, is essential for your health.

3. This generalist must be, if anything, more competent in his over-all field than a specialist, for the generalist has the ultimate responsibility for you, and he or she is the one you must rely upon to help you avoid such problems as the cases cited and to keep you in good health.

4. There are specialists whose expertise lies in being generalists and family doctors, and who can provide you with all-around care: the F.P., the general internist, the gynecologist and pediatrician for special members of the family, and for the teenagers the specialist in adolescent medicine.

5. The specialist in adolescent medicine has been created because youngsters in their teens need someone who is specially trained to handle them. Here is an ideal example of the value of the new F.P., for he can provide an ideal continuum of health care from birth through adolescence and adulthood into old age.

The next chapter will discuss how to find and check qualifications of these practitioners—the tricks of the trade, and what the expert does to solve this problem.

2

How to Find and Check a Family Doctor

It's been estimated that one in four Americans moves every year, so finding a new doctor becomes a problem for most of us sooner or later. In addition, the family doctor himself may move away, retire, or even die. The doctor's character and quality may change with time; we may become disillusioned with him. Perhaps, too, now is just the time to use the information in this book to check your current doctor's qualifications: if you find him lacking, you may want to change. Despite the number of patients concerned about or dissatisfied with physicians, there is a way to assure yourself of high-quality health and medical care. But first, why are so many people unhappy with their doctors?

"My doctor takes a quick look, grabs my money, and practically pushes me out the door," says one midwestern woman. And *Prism*, an AMA publication for doctors, relates the tale of an engineer who was called in by a doctor whose electrocardiograph was not recording the heart action of a patient. The technician came promptly. He started his check at the electrical outlet and worked back slowly to the connection to the patient in the next room—and found the patient dead. No one had even noticed that the patient's heart itself had stopped. Many find this story easy to believe from their own experiences in doctors' offices.

Many physicians have turned patients into drug addicts with improper use of narcotics, and there are many more examples of gross incompetence. An orthopedic surgeon reported at a 1973 convention that fifteen children (from one to sixteen months) suffered severe deformities as a result of improper casts for congenital dislocation of the hip.

Dr. Herbert S. Denenberg, Pennsylvania's nationally known Insurance Commissioner and consumer advocate, is concerned about authoritative claims that 5 to 15 per cent of doctors are incompetent or dishonest. As he put it recently in a speech at the University of Pennsylvania: "How would it grab you if 5 to 15 per cent of all airline pilots were incompetent or dishonest?" Makes you think, doesn't it?

Recent sociological research has revealed that medical students begin their professional schooling with idealism and humanitarianism, only to turn increasingly cynical as the four years go by. To make matters worse, there is little or no decrease in this cynicism as they move into practice. The least cynical doctors are those who go into primary care, the F.P.s or G.P.s, the internists, pediatricians, psychiatrists, and gynecologists-obstetricians. Don't these findings strengthen the reason for you to seek a generalist for your health care?

The Importance of a Good Fit

Today's patient has often read of miracle drugs, of the wonders of surgery and transplants, of heart-lung machines and artificial kidneys. But the true magic of medicine lies elsewhere, as Hippocrates, the father of medicine, well knew twenty-five hundred years ago. It lies in the doctor-patient relationship. Dr. Michael Balint, a British psychiatrist, points out in his classic book, *The Doctor, His Patient and the Illness*, that a study of the medications used most commonly by physicians revealed that "... by far the most frequently used drug in general practice was the doctor himself. ..." As Hippocrates put it, the art of medicine consists of three things: the disease, the patient, and the physician.

The doctor-patient relationship is really the key to all success in healing. Dr. Brian Bird, professor of psychiatry at Case Western Reserve, tells the story of the woman who was awaiting very dangerous surgery and was too nervous to hear the reassurances offered by the hospital doctors. Suddenly the great surgeon entered, with his staff trailing behind. Walking directly to her, he introduced himself and, shaking hands, said she looked scared to death. She burst out crying, and he simply put his arm around her for a full minute. Nothing was said, and then, with a smile and a remark that he'd see her in the morning, he left. Relaxed, she could now hear what the doctors had been trying to tell her.

In this doctor-patient relationship also lies the success of the placebo (sugar pill), which in its way is as powerful as that drug called "doctor." Any good doctor can control most pain without narcotics, given the right relationship; without a good relationship, no doctor and no drugs can control any pain.

Clearly, your hope for good health care lies in the doctor you choose. There are really two key elements: the physician must be competent and proficient in his profession; and there must be a good "fit" between patient and doctor. They must like each other, be comfortable with each other, and the patient must have faith in the doctor. Without that fit, there is virtually nothing a doctor can do to help.

Half this relationship is you. Like John in the beginning of the last chapter, you may want a doctor to simply tell you what to do, with no explanations; you may not want to share in any decisions. On the other hand, you may be like George, who was furious with a similar situation: "Doctors get me so damn mad! They try to treat you like an idiot child. I'm an intelligent adult and I want to know what it's all about—why I have the trouble I do, what he plans and why, what my medicine is and why he's giving it to me, what it'll do."

Of these two extremes, George's attitude is by far better and safer. The person who establishes a partnership with his doctor in his health care (we shall see how this is done later in this book) is likely to get better care in most instances, and certainly will protect himself from the incompetent or inconsiderate physician. But first of all you must locate a qualified doctor.

Ways to Find a Qualified Family Doctor

There are a number of ways to go about this, and even experts can't agree which is the most effective. Probably the best course is to try several methods and settle on the one most comfortable for you, or most appropriate to the particular time or place, since you're likely to have to repeat this process a number of times over the years. Or you may want to use all the techniques, utilizing them as back-up checks on the doctor you finally select.

The most common way people find doctors is probably also the worst: asking a friend or neighbor, perhaps the druggist or some tradesman, for a recommendation. Ruth, for example, likes to go to a doctor who's very busy because she figures that means he must be good; and Jack asks about "the most successful doctor in town."

Both approaches are wrong. The busiest doctor is often the one who's so interested in making money that he ends up too busy to give proper attention to anyone, while a less busy doctor may be deliberately keeping his practice to a level at which he feels he can render proper service to his patients (a very good sign if you *know* this to be the case). And "most successful" depends on what a person feels "success" is (having the largest house in town, the biggest practice, the most powerful or newest car, belonging to the right social club, etc.).

If you ask someone for the "best doctor" around or just for the name of a physician, the doctor may be recommended because he's a relative of the person you ask, or a friend or customer, a member of the same church or social club. So let's look for ways that will assure you of finding a doctor with worthwhile medical credentials and qualifications.

The simplest and quickest way—and one of the better methods—is to locate the largest and best hospital in town (and you should think twice about locating in any community that doesn't have at least a 200-bed hospital), and preferably a university teaching hospital. Then call the administrative office and ask for the names of doctors on their staff who will see you as your family doctor—either board-certified internists or board-certified F.P.s. Most hospitals keep a list of physicians willing to accept new patients. The names on the list are given out on a rotating basis, and you may be given three or four, or just the names of those in your section of town. As we shall see, hospital quality is roughly a matter of size; the larger the hospital, the better it and its staff are likely to be.

Another method is to ask who is the head of the department of internal medicine (or simply "medicine") or of family medicine—if it's a small hospital you might want to ask if he has his boards (board certification or at least eligibility is required in any decent-sized hospital). In looking for a doctor, take nothing for granted. Remember, *your* life or that of someone you love may be at stake one of these days. If there's no certified F.P., you'll have to use an internist for the adults, a gynecologist as well for the woman, a pediatrician for the children, and a specialist in adolescent medicine (if there's one in town) for the teenagers. And you may have to go through this checking process for each one, although if you find an internist you really like you might ask him to refer you to the others—or, conversely, if you find one of the others first, you might ask him to name an internist.

Another search method is to call a medical school if one is near, and here you would have a much better chance of finding a board-certified F.P. But the very minimum you should demand of any doctor is that he or she be on the staff of a community hospital. The larger and more important the hospital, the more demanding it is likely to be in medical qualifications for its staff members, and the better off you are. Doctors on the staff of a university teaching hospital are also qualified to teach their specialty, which gives you even greater assurance of their competence.

There are other reasons for the importance of hospital affiliation. A doctor on a hospital staff is likely to be exposed to continuing medical education, and without this he is behind the times. He also has an acquaintance with the specialists (surgeons or cardiologists, etc.) you may someday need. He sees how they work and how they treat their patients, how good they are—all of which gives you a better chance should he have to choose one for *you*. The larger the hospital, the larger the staff, and so the broader the variety of specialists among whom to choose. University teaching hospitals have specialists and sub-specialists (those who specialize in less frequent medical problems, such as rare blood vessel conditions or special heart x-ray techniques). Thus you would have the finest and most specialized help should a complex life-threatening medical problem arise.

Some unique and original ways of locating a physician have been suggested by Dr. John H. Knowles, former director of Massachusetts General Hospital and now president of the Rockefeller Foundation. This former specialist and medical researcher, a frank and open critic of his own profession, suggests that when you are new in town you should find a doctor by attacking the problem head on: go to the largest local hospital, get to know one of the floor nurses, and ask her who the best doctors in the hospital are, the ones most personally involved and sensitive to their patients, the ones who work the hardest and really see their patients, who respond when they are called for. Nurses will often have the best picture of what physicians are like. If necessary, ask a druggist or lawyer or banker for the name of a floor nurse and give her a ring.

Another approach is to find out who takes care of the president of your company or of the head of a big labor union and go see that doctor. But instead of contracting with him, ask who takes care of *his* family, because he certainly is in the best possible position to evaluate the physicians in his own community. Then you can double back and check these names with the local hospital nurses.

It helps, too, if one of the local medical specialists is a friend or a member of your golf club, for you can ask him the name of his family physician, or ask his opinion of the doctor whose name you've already been given.

Now, presumably, you've got enough names to choose from, so you're ready for the next step.

The First Visit: What to See and What to Ask

This is crucial, for now you must find out if there's a proper fit between you and the new doctor. Are you both in agreement that he is to run the show and you don't want to be involved in any decisions? Or do you want to share responsibility for your health care and for all necessary decisions with your new doctor? And does the doctor agree to your involvement?

You're now sitting across the desk from your new physician. Keep your eyes open. Look at the diplomas on the walls. They'll tell you if the man is a board-certified internist or F.P., and how long he's been in practice (twenty years promises sufficient experience, thirty years is excellent). If he is board-certified and the fit between you is good, you'll now want to find out:

• "If I need surgery, which surgeon would you use, Doctor?" With this name you once more make your rounds to check the surgeon. In what hospitals does he operate? What is his rank? Does he have his boards? (The next chapter will tell you how to check his hospital and what this means; Chapter 4 has more information on surgeons.) This will tell you about *your* doctor—good doctors don't refer to incompetents.

• "If I have to go into a hospital, which one would you use?" (Our next chapter will tell you about the choice of hospitals and what this says about your doctor.)

• "If there are major medical or surgical decisions to be made, do you usually get a consultation?" This is a key question, and you have to watch the physician's reaction closely. If his spine stiffens and he replies, "I don't have to get consultations, I make my own decisions," it's time to start your hunt for a family doctor again. If the answer is, "Of course, extra heads are always useful and essential—my job is to coordinate the specialists' thinking for you, to be your advocate on the health team," then you really only have a single further question to ask.

• "Do you get much of a chance to take any courses these days?" Asked innocently, this hopefully will get the truth. If he says, "I'm so busy I haven't had a chance to take a course in five years," reach for your hat. If he tells you he insists on taking time off each year to attend post-graduate courses or other continuing education, then you can relax. You've got yourself a good doctor, and you're lucky—he may save your life someday.

Of course, you may have to spread some of these questions across a couple of visits. But if you have the right doctor you can be frank and ask right off. This is itself a good sign because, above all, it's important to be able to say what you feel to your doctor.

Hospital and Medical-School Rank

Rank and titles in hospital and medical school indicate something about a doctor but not a great deal. As we have already seen, it's essential that the physician be on the staff of a good hospital, preferably the biggest in your community and connected with a university, because here other doctors are looking over his shoulder. It's been shown that board-certified physicians don't do as good a job in smaller hospitals as these same men do in university teaching hospitals.

Hospital titles and ranks vary so widely in different institutions that it's pointless to try to be too specific. A so-called attending surgeon or physician is at least one of the top men in his department, and one of these is usually the chief. "Associate attending" comes next, and then "assistant attending," but even these vary (New York's famed Memorial Sloan-Kettering Cancer Center, for example, has both a chairman and chief of anesthesiology).

In medical schools there is the head (chairman) of the department, and each department may have several full professors, along with others called "clinical professors." The only real difference here is that a full professor makes his living from his salary, while the clinical professor depends on his private practice. The "professor emeritus" is usually past sixty-five or retirement age.

Being on the staff of a hospital helps keep a doctor open to learning opportunities and provides the stimulus of interaction with other professional colleagues in both his own field and others. It gives him opportunities to meet and observe the specialists he will use for consultation, to judge both their knowledge and the way they treat their patients, as well as the interest and consideration they show their cases. Such personal contact becomes invaluable if your physician needs to refer you to a specialist. You will get more consideration and better medical care if your doctor can call the specialist and communicate directly with him, and ask him for advice and personal comments as your case progresses.

How the Internist
and Pediatrician Have Changed

Originally intended as specialists to whom their professional colleagues referred problems, the internist and the pediatrician have, like the generalist, come full circle. A recent study has revealed that the American internist actually gets fewer than one-quarter of his patients from the referrals of other physicians. Americans have increasingly discovered the internist as a generalist, and with the disappearance of the traditional family doctor this trend has accelerated.

The same thing has happened to the pediatrician. Recent figures reveal that less than one-eighth of his patients come from other doctors. Since the adults in a family have an internist as their personal physician, they need a pediatrician for the children. Confirming the widespread use of specialists instead of generalists, another recent study has revealed that New York City pediatricians spent over half their time providing well-child care, a type of practice made to order for the F.P. and really a waste of the time of a highly trained specialist. The F.P. hopefully will reverse this trend, allowing the internist and pediatrician to return to their specialties while the F.P. assumes the on-going care of the entire family.

Points to Remember

1. The key to your health care is your personal physician. He or she will be vital to your future well-being.

2. The essential factor in choosing your personal physician is "fit"—how well you two agree on the degree to which you will participate in your health-care decisions. To help you, your physician must have your respect and confidence; you must be comfortable with each other and like each other.

3. Asking a friend or other layman for a doctor is the wrong way to find a good family doctor. How busy or how "successful" he is will reveal nothing about a doctor's ability or competence—or whether he's right for *you*.

4. Your family doctor should be a board-certified internist or F.P. if you want the best possible health care.

5. Here are a number of ways to find competent practitioners: call your largest local hospital and ask for board-certified internists or F.P.s on its staff, even for the heads of these departments; contact a floor nurse at the largest hospital and ask her for the best doctors; contact the physician for your company president or union leader and ask who cares for *his* family; cross-check your findings with one other source and with any local medical specialist who may be your friend.

6. On your first visit with this prospective family doctor, look at the diplomas to be sure he is board-certified. Be certain that at the very minimum he's on the staff of one of the larger hospitals in the community, preferably a university teaching hospital. Question him to see how ready he is to call in consultants, and ask what surgeon he would use for you. Try to find out if he keeps up to date with the continuing education courses now available to all doctors.

7. Hospital and medical-school rank are so individual to the particular institution that they are meaningful only in the broadest terms.

And now for the closely related problem of finding the best hospital in the community, or checking the one that has been recommended to you.

3

Finding and Using
the Right Hospital

If you live to the Biblical three score and ten years, you're statistically likely to find yourself in a hospital a dozen times. About one in every six Americans (some 35 million of us) will be admitted to a hospital for some form of medical or surgical care this year alone, and almost half (some 12 to 15 million) will undergo surgery. The lucky ones will be healed or helped and will come out able to resume their normal lives. The unlucky, the unknowing or ignorant ones—some 100,000 or more by certain estimates—will lose their lives in that hospital, not because of surgery or the disease that brought them there but because of what happens to them in that hospital. The monetary cost too may be astronomical. One midwestern patient ran up a bill of nearly $7,500 in a mere twenty-nine hours in a hospital (the original admission was for a purely local problem). The nationwide cost of hospital-produced problems may well run close to $20 billion!

Problems You May Face in a Hospital

We're a long way from the nearly 25 per cent death rate of the Paris hospital of some two hundred years ago, when infection was virtually the norm. Still, hospital-acquired infection is probably our greatest communicable-disease problem, despite all we've learned about sterility and antibiotics. No one knows how widespread these infections are or how many people die from them. The Blue Cross magazine *Perspective* recently quoted one expert as estimating that there could be as many as 100,000 such deaths a year. The infection rate is hard to measure, and some guesses run as high as one in every six hospital patients.

There may be thousands (some have said 5,000, others two or more times that figure) of hospital patients electrocuted every year. Tiny electrical currents, so small it would take a thousand times their strength to light the smallest incandescent bulb, can throw a susceptible heart into disorganized runaway beating, which leads to death—and often a misdiagnosis of heart attack. With today's hospitals almost totally dependent on electricity, there are innumerable opportunities for defective electronic equipment to cause damage. Checks have shown that as much as half the new equipment coming into hospitals is defective—defibrillators that could kill both patient and doctor if used as delivered, defective anesthesia machines, and even such simple things as poorly designed lamps that are electrical hazards.

Then there are the dangers of simple mechanical defects—structural failures of operating and x-ray tables, litters and wheelchairs that can cause broken bones, lacerations, or bad bruises. With the increasing complexity of medical devices there is a growing number of possible failures—after all, there are now tens of thousands of medical devices, from electrocardiographs to electronic thermometers.

Just as serious a problem arises from inaccurately calibrated equipment, which may give incorrect readings and indicate medical conditions not present, or fail to reveal existing problems. To prevent instrument failure, hospitals must have engineers to set up regular examination and maintenance programs. A machine that is accurate and safe today may not be reliable tomorrow.

In New York City, one of the great meccas of medical and surgical facilities and expertise, a recent survey showed that almost 40 per cent of the hospitals should be closed down. Only one in ten had x-ray diagnostic facilities that were "reasonably adequate" (some even had to limit the number of x-rays taken for medical and surgical procedures); only one out of five surgical suites was "reasonably adequate" (counting only such gross violations as surgeons and nurses, attired in their sterile operating gowns, walking through public halls to reach the operating suite);

fewer than one out of five were in "substantial compliance" with Public Health Service fire-safety regulations. In one of the second-rank hospitals (the first are the university teaching hospitals) the surgeons felt certain that sooner or later a patient would die because the blood bank was too far from the operating-room to fill sudden surgical demands.

In mid-1973 experts concluded that a considerable portion of the surgery performed on blood vessels in the United States was unsatisfactory. Many of the nearly 75,000 reconstructions of major arteries were carried out in hospitals where fewer than 10 such operations were performed a year—but 60 or 70 must be done annually to maintain the highest quality. Specialists at Buffalo's Roswell Park Memorial Institute found that the success of radiotherapy for cancer of the uterine cervix also depended on the hospital activity: specialized cancer institutions obtained a survival rate over 50 per cent higher than that in general community hospitals. And the last few weeks of 1973 found a report in the *Journal of the American Medical Association (JAMA)* on kidney transplants: "Patient mortality at small centers is virtually double the mortality at large centers," according to the American College of Surgeons, Organ Transplant Registry. Constant practice can be translated into success, and limited experience into failure.

But what of the hospitals—how can you tell them apart, where can you get the best care, how can you use them to check the qualifications of your own doctor, how can you deal with them to get the best possible help? Here too you're faced with the tragic contrasts of American medicine, the difference between promise and realization, between triumph and tragedy, between what is possible and what is available.

Knowing Your Hospitals

America's hospitals are as diverse as the country itself, and for much the same reasons. Most obvious, of course, is the variation in size, from Alaska's 5- and 10-bed hospitals to the great metropolitan centers of the continental United States with their giant medical centers, some with 2,000 and more beds. The hospitals vary from specialty (mental or pediatric or whatever) to general; they may be voluntary or proprietary or governmental, university teaching or community. They may be called "general hospitals" or "medical centers" or just plain "hospitals." You must know what all these terms mean, particularly if you're moving into a new community or passing through an unfamiliar area. One young couple was on vacation recently when their three-year-old son developed a form of croup that suddenly choked off his breathing, turning him blue and comatose. The right hospital in that small midwest community saved the youngster's life with surgery (more on how to get help in medical emergencies in Chapter 5).

There are roughly 7,000 hospitals in the United States. Some 5,000 of these are non-governmental, the ones to which you will usually turn except in accidents or emergencies. The specialty hospitals are disappearing, which is all to the good because unless these institutions are close to general hospitals they aren't equipped to provide the broad-based, over-all services so essential to your well-being.

When Is a Hospital a Hospital —or a Medical Center?

A "medical center" can be anything from the giant hospital complex of a medical school, like New York's great Columbia-Presbyterian Medical Center, with its nearly 2,000 beds, to small hospitals with as few as 200 beds. And these simple "hospitals" too may vary from the great famous hospitals of the world (Massachusetts General Hospital) with more than 1,000 beds, down to facilities with as few as 5 beds.

The Types of Hospitals

Hospitals are classified according to their sponsorship. Federally sponsored hospitals vary from military and Veterans Administration facilities to institutes for lepers or narcotic addicts, Indians or Alaskan natives, or federal employees injured on the job. Then there are the municipal, county, district, and state hospitals.

If you need help for an acute general problem—a heart attack, special diagnostic tests, gall-bladder surgery, a delivery, or whatever—your family doctor will almost surely send you to a private hospital, usually one with which he is connected. This is why we emphasized earlier that hospital affiliation is a minimum qualification for your private physician; otherwise your case must be transferred while you're in the hospital to another doctor who's "on the staff."

There are two types of private general-care hospitals. One of the main differences between them is in their finances. The voluntary hospital is a non-profit-making corporation that pays no taxes, while the proprietary hospital is a profit-making institution and does pay taxes. Voluntary hospitals range in size and quality from such giants as Michigan's University Hospital in Ann Arbor, Baltimore's Johns Hopkins, and New York's Mount Sinai all the way down to the smallest hospital with only a handful of beds.

Proprietary hospitals also differ from voluntary hospitals in origin, purpose, and, most particularly, in quality. These hospitals can be very important in certain areas where a population explosion without a compensating growth of voluntary hospitals has created a shortage. Back in the 1930s proprietary hospitals were organized to provide a place for doctors to work (which really is what hospitals are all about) and not necessarily as just a means for making money.

Today, a doctor with a financial investment in a proprietary hospital has a divided loyalty. Realizing a profit from his patient's continued stay in his hospital as well as from his services to that patient, a physician may be tempted to hospitalize patients unnecessarily and then keep them there longer than needed so that his hospital is kept filled and profitable. Moreover, such hospitals attract doctors who do not have the professional qualifications to get on the staffs of the better hospitals. As a result, lower medical standards prevail.

In some of the voluntary giants, such as New York's Mount Sinai, there is such demand for beds that except for urgent problems (good hospitals always find a bed for any really serious problem) doctors often can't get patients in when they wish to. Thus doctors may utilize small voluntary or even good proprietary hospitals (some do have high standards) for procedures that they feel do not demand the facilities, expertise, and excellence of a Johns Hopkins or a Massachusetts General—such operations perhaps as minor skin surgery or even a "simple" gall-bladder removal. But there is always the danger of an unpredictable complication, and this is when the back-up of the major hospital can mean lives saved—or lost. One physician had his appendix removed in a small 200-bed hospital some forty miles from one of our great East Coast cities. The resulting complications almost cost him his life, and he still wonders if that forty-mile trip wouldn't have spared him all he suffered.

Proprietary hospitals are definitely disappearing from the national scene; in the decades to come you very likely won't have to worry about them. But here too the selection of your family doctor is all-important. An honest, competent, concerned physician is your best protection against the wrong hospital.

Where Can You Check Your Hospital?

If you want to check whether a hospital is proprietary, how large it is, what services it offers, how active it is in the form of surgery you need, your best bet is, first, your family doctor (assuming he's both competent and concerned with you). You may also go to your library and consult the annual guide put out by the AHA (American Hospital Association). Each year this magazine seems to change its cover and its name: it may be the "Guide Issue" of the AHA publication *Hospitals;* it may be in one part or two; or it may simply be *The AHA Guide to the Health Care Field*—your librarian should be able to help. A small library may not have this volume, and you may have to turn to a college or university or medical society library. This publication, however, covers virtually everything—all hospitals, their type, their facilities, how many beds they have, and so on.

Another excellent source of information, at least in the larger urban centers, is the Health and Hospital (or just plain Hospital) Planning Council, a quasi-official agency that can offer information of enormous value in your quest for better health care. A telephone call to the nearest one (city, county, or state) will quickly get you details on the available hospital facilities in your locality.

When a Bed Is More Than a Bed

Since a hospital room may contain two or more beds, the number of rooms in a hospital would be meaningless. "Bed" figures immediately indicate how many patients can be accommodated (they actually ran about 80 per cent occupied in 1971). The larger hospitals with their 1,000 and more beds are giant institutions—for instance, Los Angeles County–University of Southern California Medical Center has 2,100 beds and employs 7,300 people (not counting interns, residents, nurses, or volunteers).

The importance of the number of beds is simply that the larger hospitals are likely to provide better medical and surgical care. They can afford to have more sophisticated and more specialized equipment. They usually have bigger medical staffs with doctors skilled not only in the major specialties, such as neurology and radiology, but even in the infrequently used sub-specialties (rare diseases, head and heart x-rays, nuclear medicine).

What size should be minimal? This depends in part on geography. In thinly populated states like Alaska and Idaho, small hospitals of 20, 50, or 100 beds are essential. They provide immediate medical and surgical care and save the sick person from traveling hundreds of miles to a larger city, which may still have only a 200- or 250-bed hospital with limited staff and facilities as compared to the urban giants.

You might well seek a 400- to 500-bed hospital. The Southern New York Health and Hospital Planning Council has set 400 beds as New York City's minimum. In fact, you would certainly not be unreasonable if you hesitated to move to any community without at least a 350-bed hospital. You need only look at the *AHA Guide* to realize how vastly the facilities of a 1,000-bed hospital outrank those of a 400-bed hospital, and how vastly this in turn outranks a 200-bed hospital. Of course, some small hospitals are magnificently equipped, such as the Hunterdon Medical Center of Flemington, New Jersey, or some of the small Kaiser Foundation Hospitals in California, but these are definitely the rare exceptions.

Accreditation and Affiliation:
Who Rates Your Hospital?

State agencies (usually the departments of public health) periodically check certain aspects of hospitals, such as the safety of x-ray machines, but these examinations vary widely in their efficiency and meaningfulness. The Joint Commission on Hospital Accreditation (JCAH) was formed by the AHA, AMA, and the American Colleges of Physicians and of Surgeons. It inspects hospitals on a voluntary basis every two years, but it has been accused of paying attention only to the quality of record-care and not to patient-care. Actually, checking JCAH accreditation is like checking that your family doctor is on the staff of a hospital—both are the barest minimum qualifications. While JCAH accreditation guarantees virtually nothing as to the quality of patient-care, if a hospital does *not* have it, you're probably best off staying away.

What *is* meaningful in the way of formal qualifications? For one thing, the hospital's affiliations are important. Is the hospital a university teaching hospital, or the chief hospital for a university medical school, such as Massachusetts General, Harvard, Cornell? These hospitals are staffed by the medical schools, which provide their own teachers as the doctors of the hospitals, thus assuring the latest in knowledge and techniques. True, you may have to put up with young medical students, residents, or interns trailing around listening to your doctor's explanation of your case, but it's well worth the nuisance to secure the best available medical and surgical know-how.

Next best are the affiliated hospitals, which have looser connections to medical schools. Here the hospital may or may not be fully staffed by the medical school, but there are various degrees of overlapping. The so-called "teaching" hospitals come next, but this term is as untrustworthy as "medical center." It may indicate that the hospital has a program to train interns and residents, an affiliated nursing school, or just a school for some sort of medical technician. You must find out what "teaching" really means before you can make any decision about a teaching hospital.

Lowest on the totem pole is the unaffiliated and non-teaching hospital, the one with virtually no qualifications. These of course must be judged in the light of geography. If there are no medical schools or universities anywhere around, you can't expect a hospital to create one.

Some Ways the Experts Use
to Evaluate Hospitals

House staff. These are the interns and residents (young doctors learning a specialty), and in the United States today there are more positions available than young doctors to fill them. Active internship and residency programs indicate that the hospital is accredited by the AMA or by specialty organizations for advanced training of young doctors—a sign of quality medical care. A large number of vacancies in a house staff may well mean that a poor reputation is causing young doctors to avoid the hospital; a full staff of American-trained young physicians shows that recent graduates have been given good reports of the medical and surgical know-how available there.

The best index of quality hospital care. Dr. Jack C. Haldeman, president of the Health and Hospital Review and Planning Council of Southern New York and former chief of the Division of Hospital and Medical Facilities of the United States Public Health Service, believes the best index is the percentage of foreign medical-school graduates (FMG) on the house staff. Coming in with language difficulties and trained in foreign medical schools, which might well be sub-standard, a high percentage of FMGs may well be an indication that the institution is not good or that American graduates are avoiding it. But a lack of house staff may even sometimes be a plus. One surgical patient became very ill following an operation at a small hospital that had no FMGs, interns, or residents. His surgeon slept at the hospital for two nights during the critical illness, giving him better service than he would have had at a larger hospital staffed with FMGs.

Empty beds. A hospital with a lot of empty beds is one to avoid. It may be pressuring physicians on its staff to bring in patients to fill those empty beds or to keep patients longer than necessary to keep up occupancy.

Average length of stay of patients. This figure may be difficult to find and is tricky to evaluate, since a high proportion of elderly patients may shoot it above average. Usually, though, the shorter the stay, the more careful the hospital is in its bed utilization, and so the more efficient. Also, a short average length of stay may indicate that the hospital is staffed with the new breed of surgeons who like to see their patients go home as soon as possible after an operation.

Autopsy rate. If you call the hospital's pathology laboratory, you may be able to find their autopsy percentage. Where this is high, it indicates a hospital with enough concern for its patients so that it constantly desires to find out the facts of a case.

Consultations. If you have a chance to observe the hospital in action, watch how often several doctors cluster together to examine a patient or discuss a chart. Consultations show concern for patients, and it's been said that consultations could be of advantage to as many as one out of every five patients in any general hospital.

Staff qualifications. You should certainly try to learn whether the specialists and heads of departments are required to be board-certified, and whether surgeons without board certification are allowed to operate there. The percentage of staff that is board-certified or board-eligible is another good indication of the quality of a hospital.

Hospital services. Your hospital should have a broad range of services, with board-certified internists, surgeons, neurologists, psychiatrists, pediatricians, obstetrician-gynecologists, radiologists (x-ray specialists), pathologists (to examine tissues microscopically and perform other laboratory functions), anesthesiologists, urologists, and ophthalmologists available if not on staff. Also important are necessary back-up services: a general intensive-care unit, a coronary-care unit, histopathology laboratory, post-operative recovery room, a blood bank, and preferably an emergency department staffed (as we shall see in Chapter 5) by full-time personnel.

Points to Remember

1. Your hospital should preferably be a voluntary (not proprietary) university teaching hospital or one affiliated with a medical school, of at least 400 to 500 beds if possible; JCAH accreditation is a basic minimum.

2. American interns and residents filling all openings is a good

sign, as is an active intern and residency program. A large proportion of foreign medical-school graduates as interns and residents is a bad sign, as are large numbers of vacancies in the house staff.

3. Empty beds in large numbers and a long average length of stay should make one suspect a hospital's quality.

4. A high percentage of board-certified people as specialists, surgeons, and heads of departments shows quality care. A high percentage of autopsies is another good sign.

5. A wide range of hospital services should be available.

6. The *AHA Guide* is invaluable for checking many of these questions, as is the local Health and Hospital Planning Council.

4
Surgery Can Be Murder:
How to Protect Yourself

Helen froze in horror as the surgeon picked up his phone, saying, "I want to call the hospital to make arrangements for immediate surgery for that lump. If the entire breast has to be removed the fee will be . . ." By now Helen was too shocked to hear the rest of what the surgeon said. Meanwhile Morton was told, "You have a hernia which should be operated on promptly. How soon can you enter the hospital?" And Bob, who suffered some winter sore throats, was advised by his doctor to have his tonsils removed.

Helen had this experience in New York, while the two men had theirs in different large cities west of the Mississippi. None of these operations has yet been performed—or ever will be, because Helen, Morton, and Bob knew what to do when faced with suggested surgery.

These were three of the many thousands of unnecessary operations advised and often carried out every year. This chapter can help *you* protect your life and health from unscrupulous, mistaken, or knife-happy surgeons.

According to the *New York Times,* one doctor recently admitted to performing nearly forty unnecessary operations. Such surgeons cause the deaths of perhaps tens of thousands of Americans annually, and when a patient dies from an unnecessary operation it's just plain murder.

No one can ever know for sure how a patient will react to any anesthetic or surgical procedure. There will always be unavoidable deaths (one figure commonly mentioned is 1.2 per cent), but there should be no blame when the surgery has been done for good reasons by a competent surgeon in an adequate hospital. When an attempt is made to save a person's life through surgery, the necessary risk is worthwhile.

But what justification can there be when a patient dies from an unnecessary operation, and the surgeon knows it's the procedure often referred to in doctors' locker rooms as "acute remunerative appendicitis"? Or when the operation falls into the class of such medical wisecracks as "When in doubt take it out," or "Everybody has three or more surgical problems—all you have to do is to locate them"? There are 14 million (some say 20 million) operations performed every year in the United States, and evidence indicates that from 20 to 60 per cent of these are unnecessary! Since the death rate from surgery over-all is commonly put at 1.2 per cent, it would seem that tens of thousands of patients die unnecessarily from surgery.

There are many concerned physicians, and some have even carried their messages directly to the public in an attempt to correct this abuse. Others will talk of the subject anonymously, in private. One young neurologist in a well-known western medical center told me of the heart surgeon in his hospital who remarked he'd just done an appendectomy. When the young man looked aghast (especially in surgery, the specialist should stick to his field), the surgeon laughed. "Don't you know I'm a hand surgeon?" Then he explained, "I do anything I can get my hands on." And on the East Coast a chest surgeon in a large hospital boasted to a medical colleague that he'd done hundreds of hysterectomies in a small proprietary hospital in the same community.

Not surprisingly, surgeons are hit with more than half the malpractice suits brought against doctors, and the news media can testify to the extent of the problem. One surgeon placed an unnecessarily tight cast on a patient's broken leg, causing gangrene and, in the end, amputation; another patient's leg was amputated for a cancer that wasn't there. The Commission on Medical Malpractice recently found insurance carriers themselves admitting that virtually half (46 per cent) of patients' claims were "meritorious."

Unnecessary operations range all the way from the downright bizarre to the simple abuse of common procedures. Dr. Walter Alvarez, professor emeritus of the Mayo Graduate School of Medicine, tells of more than a hundred hysterectomies done to relieve migraine. Large numbers of tonsils and adenoids are being removed; a seemingly simple operation, it nevertheless takes the lives of several hundred children every year and may expose the others to serious diseases later in life.

In surgery too there is that contrast between the miracles that are possible and the needless death, suffering, and economic loss that all too frequently occur. Yet many patients actually seek operations, and they can always find a doctor to oblige. If you decide you need surgery (even though you really don't), you're likely to end up with it.

The Dollars and Cents of This Problem

The surgeon too wants to feed his family, buy his wife a mink coat, send his children to college, have two cars in his garage, and indulge his hobbies. To accomplish all this in our fee-for-service medical system, he has to perform operations—and the United States has simply turned out too many surgeons. The latest figures show that the qualified American surgeon performs an average of only 3.8 operations (major *and* minor) a week, about half what his British counterpart does. In short, our surgeons are being over-produced and underworked.

To make matters worse, American surgeons are being turned out at a faster rate than our population growth. October 1973 saw the largest group of young surgeons in history recognized as specialists—1,675 became Fellows of the American College of Surgeons (F.A.C.S. is what they'll put after their names and their M.D.s)—and this is important for you to remember and recognize, because it promises you that the F.A.C.S. doctor is a properly trained surgeon.

Since he does piecework, getting paid for what he turns out, the surgeon is under personal and economic pressure to operate, and this push may even come from his hospital. The large university teaching hospitals are usually so busy that they permit their surgeons only a limited number of "elective" operations (those whose need and time are by choice, like most varicose vein removals); but a smaller hospital may pressure its surgeons to operate more, to fill its beds and utilize its operating facilities.

What's Going on Here?

Study after study shows that the amount of surgery grows in proportion to the numbers of surgeons and hospital beds available. For example, in England and Wales, with half the number proportionately of our surgeons, half as many or fewer operations are performed than in the United States—but no one has ever suggested that insufficient surgery is being done in Britain.

Dr. John P. Bunker, professor of anesthesia at Stanford University—along with many other experts—feels that we have too many surgeons. Almost half (40 per cent) of all our young doctors in residency (specialty) training are in general surgery or in some surgical specialty.

Repeated studies both here and abroad have shown that the number of appendectomies, gall-bladder operations, hernia repairs, and tonsillectomies varies directly with the facilities and manpower available. Dr. Charles E. Lewis, professor of preventive medicine at the University of California, at Los Angeles, has shown that even within a single state the frequency of these operations can run three to four times as high in some regions as in others —and this rate varies directly with the numbers of surgeons and of hospital beds.

The Numbers and Quality of Surgeons

The United States certainly has the numbers: there are more neurosurgeons in Massachusetts than in all of England and Wales (with eleven times that commonwealth's population); more chest surgeons were certified in the United States in 1971 alone than all such surgeons practicing in England and Wales.

Quality is another story, and in surgery that is usually measured by who does the operations. Where in England and Wales and Sweden (to name another country), only recognized specialists are allowed to operate, here in the United States nearly half our surgery is done by non-certified surgeons. In short, you must be doubly alert if you are to protect yourself.

Who Should Perform the Surgery?

As with a family doctor, you want someone with board certification, and in surgery this is even more important, for your life is on the line every time you undergo surgery. So too is your well-being. Dr. Theodore Rubin, a well-known psychiatrist and author, tells how, at the hospital where he interned, a neurosurgeon condemned a seventeen-year-old boy to a lifetime of paraplegia by cutting the lad's spinal cord during surgery.

That a doctor has his boards in surgery and is an F.A.C.S. (not the same and both should be there) is no guarantee of ability, but they do indicate that the doctor has been trained properly, and these qualifications should be the minimum. There are still occasional doctors who, without these credentials, are competent surgeons, but to use such a person is too risky—unless it's an emergency in a remote area where no one else is available.

Another good sign is that the surgeon is on the staff of one of the best, and largest, hospitals in your community. As we have mentioned before, a university teaching hospital is ideal because so many professional colleagues look over the surgeon's shoulder. A surgeon who has an appointment only in a proprietary hospital is not a good risk, although many excellent surgeons do operate in these and other small hospitals because they can't get much of their elective surgery into the large ones.

Age too is considered a factor by many experts, who won't recommend a surgeon over sixty-five unless they personally know that the person is skillful. Surgery is a hard life, and it takes a lot of stamina to stand and work at an operating table for four hours or more at a stretch.

Where Should You Start the Road to Surgery?

Certainly, do not start with a surgeon, for his whole training and philosophy is that of the operating room, of cutting out disease with a knife. Moreover, technical skills, learning to be a good carpenter, as it were, are a lot simpler and so more common than the subtle art of diagnosis, which tells when to operate and when not to.

Clearly, the good family doctor is your first line of defense against unnecessary surgery and should be consulted initially. As we've already seen, the American surgeon is underworked and has a vested interest in performing surgery. With the best will in the world, it's too easy for any human being to rationalize that the procedures he wants to perform and has been highly trained to carry out are the ones that should be done.

Fee-Splitting and Ghost Surgery: Twin Menaces

If you find your family doctor is to receive a fee in connection with your operation (whether for "assisting" or whatever), you have good reason to suspect fee-splitting and to seek other doctors. Although the chances of fee-splitting are minimized by consultations, as we shall see later, the danger of this practice is that your family doctor may acquire a vested interest in your undergoing surgery.

Thus, one of the dangers of proprietary hospitals is that both family doctor and surgeon (anyone who has a share in the hospital) have a vested interest in your undergoing an operation—fee-splitting, as it were, with a hospital instead of just with another doctor.

Ghost surgery is at least as bad and even more directly dangerous. In this, the supposed surgeon is in the operating room, but once the patient is unconscious the "ghost" takes over the operation. The dangers here are manifold. The decision to operate is made by the "front" surgeon, probably no more competent in his diagnosis than in his surgery, increasing the likelihood of unnecessary or misdirected surgery. The "ghost" is commonly a young, inexperienced, or not too competent surgeon who has no adequate practice of his own. Finally, the "ghost"—the only one who knows anything, little as that may be—has no responsibility after the operation when complications may well threaten or even cost the life of the patient.

This practice goes on even in our better hospitals because doctors are notoriously unwilling—out of friendship or pity or camaraderie or whatever—to take operating privileges away from their fellow doctors. In one of the large university teaching hospitals on the East Coast, one surgeon was in his eighties before he stopped (on his own) "operating." Actually, his residents had been doing his surgery for a long time, but no one tried to stop him. Nevertheless, the better the hospital, the better your protection —all things being equal.

In short, you have to rely on yourself. Here are some of the ways in which you can protect yourself when you have been told you need surgery.

What to Look for in a Surgeon

Obviously the first thing is to check in your library (we've detailed this in the chapter on your family doctor) to be sure that he is board-certified and an F.A.C.S., that he is on the staff of a reputable hospital. You can also see how old he is, how long he's been in practice, what hospital rank he holds, and whether he teaches in a medical school. You can interpret all of this in conjunction with our earlier chapters.

You should be especially careful of the surgeon's age. He should not, in general, be over sixty-five; nor should he be too young. While a very young man can be an excellent technician (some teachers claim they can train virtually anyone in a year's time to be an excellent surgeon technically, to cut and splice and so on), the fine diagnostic abilities, the discrimination and knowledge, take many years of experience to reach their peak.

How to Choose Your Surgeon

Recommendations by knowledgeable people—your family doctor, a hospital nurse familiar with his work, other doctors— should be used in choosing the surgeon. His credentials too must check out, as has just been discussed. And, of course, you must like your surgeon, feel comfortable with him, and have confidence in him (most surgeons are men today, but this will surely change).

Another helpful method is to ask the people from whom you seek a referral to name three surgeons in order of their preference, then compare the lists and start with the one who is on top or close to it most often. One of the very best recommendations is that a doctor you respect used the surgeon for himself or his family. Then you must meet the doctor and take one final major consideration into account.

Consultation: Test and Protection

The key to better surgical care is to ask for a consultation, which will tell you a lot and protect your life and limb. Before undergoing any surgery, except for the most urgent case (severe injury or whatever), it is absolutely essential *to have at least one independent consultation.* (The "independent" here is important too.) Actual trials have clearly proved that consultations have actually reduced the amount of surgery by anywhere from 20 to 60 per cent.

Tell the surgeon you initially consult that you would like a consultation (assuming he's advised surgery). If he gets his back up about this, you are probably dealing with the wrong person —although you may, on confirming his judgment, still prefer him to do your surgery. Competent surgeons who are confident of their ability and expertise will welcome consultation; for one thing, consultation reassures the patient about the surgeon's judgment and ability and leaves him more cooperative.

Ask your family doctor to suggest the second surgeon to be consulted; otherwise, you'll have to try the same method you used to find your original surgeon, or you can use the number two man from your original list. The advantage of having your family physician in on this decision or at least advised of it is that the consultant may want to speak with your doctor to get some medical information about you. In any case, the consultant should be a surgeon who doesn't know your original choice, who preferably doesn't even work at the same hospital.

Then lay it right on the line that you want only a consultation, that you've selected a surgeon but want another opinion. Then the consultant knows he's not going to be doing the surgery, so he has nothing to gain by advising an operation, which eliminates any built-in vested interest. Some people even suggest that the second consultant not know the conclusions of the first surgeon, since he may be influenced by them. But this approach does have the disadvantage of leaving him open to the thought of getting the job himself.

Two confirmatory consultations should always be considered in very serious surgical problems. Checking this way may cost you some money, but it's well worth it if you are in the 20 to 60 per cent who really *don't* need the surgery.

Some Extra Important Points on Surgeons and Surgery

It's important that the surgeon isn't too busy to give you the time and attention you should have. This is tricky to decide because the best surgeons are bound to be busy, but you can get some feel for this by the time he gives you and his willingness to explain what has to be done and why. *Always* ask about the possible problems or complications of the surgery, what other choices there are, and where you can look up information on the subject so you fully understand what's planned (see the last chapter).

The Danger Spots: Beware!

In particular, you must be on guard when the operation is one of those most often unnecessarily performed today, such as hysterectomies, mastectomies (breast removals), tonsillectomies, hemorrhoidectomies, hernia repairs, and even appendectomies (except for the truly emergency ones, of course). In "A Shopper's Guide to Surgery," Dr. Denenberg has outlined a number of ways to protect yourself. He points out that these operations have been named "remunerectomies" (a play on "remuneration"), while Dr. Norman S. Miller of the University of Michigan has coined the word "hip-pocket hysterectomies," because their beneficiary is the pocket where the surgeon keeps his wallet.

Points to Remember

1. Since 20 to 60 per cent of the surgery performed is unnecessary, much of it done by unqualified practitioners, and since many procedures being carried out are injurious, you must take every possible precaution to protect yourself.

2. A surgeon should be board-certified and an F.A.C.S. (Fellow of the American College of Surgeons) wherever possible (in remote areas, emergencies may require using whoever does the surgery there). The surgeon should also be on the staff of the best and largest hospital in your community, preferably a university teaching hospital if there is one. Certainly you should be wary of any surgeon who is *only* on the staff of a proprietary hospital. It's always a wise precaution to know if your surgery falls into the area of a surgical specialty (neurosurgery, vascular surgery, etc.) and if your surgeon specializes in it.

3. No surgery should be undergone without at least one independent consultation. The consulting surgeon should know he's not going to do the surgery, that you want only his opinion, and he should have no knowledge of or connection with the other surgeon. If two consultants are used, one might not even be told what the others have said.

4. Use your family doctor, nurses, or other doctors as sources of surgical recommendations. Draw up a list of names in the order preferred, then choose the name which comes at the top most often. This also gives you a list from which to choose another surgical consultation later on.

5. Never start the search for surgery with a surgeon, because he's much more likely to think first of cutting. A good family doctor is the best place to start.

6. Be certain that any surgeon over sixty-five years of age is particularly well known and highly regarded. Not many doctors over sixty-five can stand for four hours or more at the operating table.

7. Don't pick a surgeon who is too busy—he may not give you the time and attention you need. Find out what the possible surgical problems or complications may be, what other choices there are, and where you can get more information on your problem (see the last chapter).

8. Since surgery is a life-threatening procedure and there are so many complications and questions, it might be wise before agreeing on surgery to go over this chapter in detail.

Our next chapter, too, involves life-threatening situations—medical emergencies, how to prepare for them, and how to handle them when they occur.

5

How to Get Life-Saving Help in Medical Emergencies

An ambulance—supposedly a promise of help and safety—with its siren screaming and red overhead light flashing, raced up the driveway of a busy hospital in an Ohio city. The ambulance attendants rushed the accident victim, on a stretcher, into the emergency room. Here the doctor removed the oxygen mask from the injured person, to find it so filled with blood and vomitus that the patient couldn't breathe through it. Not long before, an unconscious patient had been brought in, suffocating, because he had been placed face down on a stretcher; while another arrived so placed that both nose and mouth were buried in blankets.

In another midwestern hospital a teenager was safely brought in after a high-speed auto accident. Since he had difficulty in breathing, the medical personnel bent the victim's neck backward to slip a tube down his throat to aid in breathing. That youngster will be a quadriplegic for the rest of his days: bending his neck completed the fracture of his spine, damaging the spinal cord irreparably. Properly trained emergency physicians would have used other methods to assist breathing, and that boy would never have been paralyzed.

But let's look also at the other side of the coin: in Jacksonville, Fla., I've personally talked with people who have died (they had no heartbeat, no pulse, no longer breathed). These people are now perfectly well and can probably look forward to whatever life span their health and age normally allow. In Michigan I spent time with a mother whose two-year-old son had developed an acute form of croup, which suddenly shut off his breathing and turned him blue-black, by the time his parents were able to get him to a hospital with highly trained emergency physicians. That lad was racing around, perfectly well, with only a tiny dimple on the front of his neck where an opening had been cut to permit insertion of a tube into his windpipe (a "tracheostomy") to make breathing possible once more. The tube remained there until the croup subsided and the swollen throat returned to normal, permitting the child to breathe once more through his mouth.

The problem of medical care in emergencies touches or threatens all of us—and the price is deadly. Every year more than 52 million Americans are injured; over 110,000 of these accident victims die, and about .5 million suffer lasting disability. Nearly 2 million children suffer accidental poisoning every year, and the resulting deaths may run into the thousands. One outstanding authority believes these poisoning figures are only the tip of the iceberg, and that many instances are not diagnosed or even reported. And, finally, nearly 750,000 Americans die each year from heart attacks, and about half of these never reach the hospital alive.

How many of these people died unnecessarily and prematurely? How many lives could have been saved by proper emergency care in time? Dr. Henry C. Huntley, Director of the United States Division of Emergency Health Services, recently estimated—on the basis of careful national studies and demonstrations—that 60,000 Americans (some experts estimate as high as 90,000) lose their lives unnecessarily every year simply because the emergency medical care they receive is inadequate. And no one even tries to estimate the amount of unnecessary permanent damage and disability that has resulted from this system. Lives are wasted simply because either equipment or personnel or expertise was lacking at the scene, in the ambulance, or in the hospital ED (emergency department).

In emergency medical care the gap between what is possible and what is actually available is certainly one of the greatest in all health care. In this chapter you will find some of the ways in which *you* can reduce or minimize this gap. The best possible emergency care is now available in the United States—but you have to know what it is, what to look for, and how to find it.

Understanding Emergency Medical Care

There is a basic change in our pattern of health care that must be understood if you're to find the best protection in an emergency. As in all medical care, there are two basic elements—equipment and personnel—and personnel is the more important, for the best equipment in the world is useless without properly trained human beings. But the concept of personnel and its uses has changed.

We've come a long way since the 1930s, when a doctor (traditionally a young intern) rode the ambulance on each call. With World War II, doctors became scarce and were too busy to make ambulance calls. The old pattern went the way of the dodo bird —and, under the proper circumstances, you're much the better for it. The physicians of the 1930s—and most of those of today—actually compare quite unfavorably with today's highly specialized and trained emergency medical technicians. These so-called EMTs ride ambulances and make them the truly life-saving vehicles they can be. And, ideally, a well-trained doctor waits within the confines of his hospital emergency department for the skilled EMTs to bring in the victims they have kept alive. The physicians can then use their own skills and all the sophisticated technology of a modern hospital to save injured and acutely ill human beings.

You have to depend on yourself to determine the value of the ambulance service and the emergency department in your area. In a recent poll, over 90 per cent of doctors thought their ambulance services were good, while only 60 per cent of the operators thought so; actually, both were outlandishly optimistic. But you have to know—it's *your* life.

Preparing Your Family for a Medical Emergency

Ideally, in an emergency you should be familiar with advanced first aid and CPR (cardiopulmonary resuscitation)—so should all adults and teenagers in the family. But let's forget the ideal and be practical, for it will be a long time before this training reaches every American, and not even doctors can be objective enough to treat their own families.

Getting emergency medical help is not as simple as it sounds, for even your family doctor (unless he's an F.P.) is not likely to be trained to carry out necessary emergency care. The new F.P.s can, but internists aren't likely to be prepared to cope with emergencies. A doctor's knowledge of emergency procedures depends on his specialty (anesthesiologists are likely to be best, and such specialists as dermatologists and psychiatrists poorest). There is a movement afoot to require annual reregistration for physicians, and some people want knowledge of CPR to be a requirement for this. But all this is in the future, perhaps far off. Besides, no patient needs to be told today how difficult it can be to reach a doctor at any time, particularly during evenings or nights, weekends or holidays.

Tragically, there is no single nationwide telephone number you can use for emergency medical help, although the 911 system is beginning to take hold. All those in the emergency field hope to see 911 used nationally some day. But right now you have to learn how to summon help in your community or vacation spot. For example, in Jacksonville, Florida, a specific widely advertised number will cut you right into the emergency health-care system, and special public telephones do the same as soon as the receiver is picked up (if you passed out, the dangling receiver would bring help automatically). At the other extreme, some communities require a police officer to be dispatched when an accident is reported. Only when he arrives at the scene and verifies the medical emergency will an ambulance be sent on its way.

The local telephone directory isn't much help, for it won't tell you what the hospital emergency departments or ambulance services are like, or how they are staffed or equipped. Ambulance services are even called by different names: they are "Rescue Squads" in Jacksonville, "Emergency Squads" in Columbus, Ohio, and "Life Squads" in Cincinnati. In some places they're not in the phone book at all.

In some communities the ambulance service is operated by the police or the fire department, and some of these—Jacksonville, Louisville, Baltimore—rank among the nation's best. The service may also be run by volunteers (many of these are of the highest caliber) or by hospitals or private companies. Actually, any particular ambulance setup may be at the top or the bottom of the ladder; you just have to be familiar with the individual situation.

It may be time to take a new look at the emergency medical setup in your own community, using the standards and questions we offer in this chapter. Certainly you must do this promptly if you move to a new community, or even if you plan to stay only a few days or weeks in a place—particularly if your family or group includes a sick person, someone with a chronic condition like asthma, which can suddenly precipitate an acute medical crisis, small children, or elderly people.

The two elements most commonly needed in any medical emergency are the ambulance service and the hospital emergency department. You should familiarize yourself with the best ones in your area (using the questions and criteria we'll shortly provide) and have their phone numbers handy. Here then is the detailed information on how to judge these services.

Is the Ambulance a Hearse?

All too often, yes, and literally! Our ambulance situation is certainly one of the most disgraceful in the whole American health-care system. Statistics show that, despite recent improvements, nearly half of our nation's ambulances are still owned and operated by funeral homes. The latest National Academy of Sciences/National Research Council (NAS/NRC) study reveals that more than four-fifths of our 25,000 ambulances are of the hearse, limousine, or station-wagon type, entirely inadequate as ambulances in both space and equipment.

Only some half of our ambulances are capable of radio communication with the dispatcher (essential for ordering and routing, when additional help or information is urgently needed, and to prepare the hospital for the patient's reception). A miniscule 6 per cent of our ambulances have the capacity—absolutely essential if lives are to be saved—to communicate directly with the emergency department of the hospital so that the doctor can supervise emergency care in serious cases. An ambulance should also be equipped to transmit electrocardiograms (EKGs) to the hospital so the physicians there can read them and advise the ambulance personnel on how to care for the patient on the way in.

Then there is the ambulance personnel. An ambulance must have both a driver and an attendant as a bare minimum, yet in Connecticut—not atypical of other states—almost 10 per cent of the ambulance services send a vehicle with only a driver. Nationwide, 10 per cent of ambulance attendants have *no* training at all, even in the fundamentals of first aid, and 33 per cent have only standard Red Cross first aid training (experts regard even advanced first aid as totally inadequate for ambulance personnel). The NAS/NRC report quotes estimates that fewer than 35 per cent of these people are qualified even at the recommended *minimal* level, which is 80 hours of training. Leading organizations in emergency health care are now calling for an additional 480-hour advanced training program and the creation of a corps of lifesaving emergency medical technicians (EMTs).

The EMT is qualified to handle virtually every emergency medical problem he or she meets up with. An EMT is a paraprofessional, able to examine a victim, determine the problem, and render immediate care to keep the patient alive and prevent further harm while transporting him to a hospital for definitive medical treatment.

Jacksonville's Rescue Squads are manned by firemen who volunteered for this duty and underwent special training, which continues throughout their service. They can safely extricate an auto-crash victim from virtually any kind of wreck (they cut the car away from the person), restore and maintain breathing and heart action, control bleeding, give intravenous and other injections, take EKGs and transmit them from their special custom-made ambulances back to the emergency department, where a doctor follows the case; they are even trained to use the defibrillator (a device whose powerful electrical shock can start a stopped heart or shock a weak, confused beat back to its normal rhythm), which is part of the equipment in their vehicle. They know how to handle any fractures—leg or spine or whatever.

What does this system mean to you, the consumer? It means medical security, safety, and added years of life. Captain John M. Waters, Jacksonville's director of public safety and one of the nation's great emergency-medical-care experts, has pointed out that in 1970 alone the city's emergency-care system was able to cut highway deaths to fewer than half those in 1969, administered CPR to 88 people, and delivered 77 of these "dead" people to the hospital alive!

How to Assure Good Ambulance Service

When you suddenly need emergency medical help you're not likely to be cool enough or have sufficient time to get proper ambulance service—unless you're fortunate enough to be in one of those widely scattered spots with good ambulance service (there's no point trying to name them, because they change with time and are, hopefully, increasing). So do it now, or when you first arrive in a new community.

The first step is to check the front of the local phone book to see if a phone number for ambulance service is listed after those for police and fire: this may be 911 (as in New York City), or a specific one, as in Jacksonville, or it may be a matter of calling the police or fire emergency number. If there is no specific ambulance number, ask the advice of an emergency physician on the staff of the community hospital—he is the person most knowledgeable about ambulance services because he works so closely with them. If an emergency physician is not available, you will have to learn to ask the right questions.

Once you've located the available facilities—many communities have a variety of ambulance services, including private, governmental (police or fire or other), and volunteer—you can ask which one handles emergencies. Some do only transportation, and the phone book usually doesn't distinguish. Then there really are only a few questions to ask:

• Does this ambulance service always respond to calls with at least an attendant and a driver? (This is essential.)

• Are all ambulance personnel EMTs? Usually such people are proud to have their EMT emblem or shield on their shoulder or chest pocket; this promises top professional competence. Although it is possible for people to be trained to this level without being EMTs, usually a person who reaches that level wants this recognition. In any case, it is essential that ambulance personnel be capable of performing CPR, dealing with medical emergencies of all types, and even extricating people from wrecks. Moreover, the service should conduct on-going training to keep up its personnel quality.

• The ambulances themselves should meet the requirements set down by the NAS/NRC (you can get a copy of these from the

United States Department of Health, Education, and Welfare or the American College of Surgeons).

• The ambulances should carry the first aid supplies and rescue and medical equipment advised by these same organizations.

• The dispatcher should be as well trained as an EMT so that he or she can understand the problem and route the calls properly.

• The ambulance should have two-way radio communications with both its dispatcher and its hospital emergency department.

Given today's state of emergency medical affairs, you may not find the ideal ambulance service. At least, think twice about settling in any community without an adequate emergency healthcare system, for such a decision might someday be worth your life.

The Help of the Future

It may be difficult for some people to accept the EMT—who may be a "she" or a "he"—as the one to perform these life-saving jobs at the scene of an emergency. But this is the way of the future—paraprofessionals are increasingly taking over many of the tasks traditionally reserved for physicians. Those who fought in our wars beginning with World War II are familiar with the life-saving the "medics" did—just as the EMTs are doing today. Sex-role concepts will also have to be shed, for women are increasingly staffing volunteer ambulance services.

But what of the hospitals and their emergency departments, the doctors who staff them, and how can you assure good emergency care at this level?

The Emergency Departments and Their Doctors

Until recently emergency rooms were dingy, poorly equipped backwaters of their hospitals, where the intern or newest staff doctor served out his term until he could pass this distasteful job on to someone else. The new crisis in medical care has changed all this. Unable to get a physician in an emergency—or an evening or holiday or weekend—Americans have turned to the hospital EDs. The old emergency room has become an up-to-date emergency department, with some 50 million patient visits in 1970 alone. Moreover, new life-saving techniques—CPR, defibrillators, and other devices—make it possible to actively preserve and even restore life.

The result has been a new breed of doctors—mostly in their forties and fifties, action-oriented, devoted to medicine—a new specialty, the "emergency physician." These doctors are trained or experienced in emergency medical care. They are not interested in medical care in depth; they seek to provide only immediate, urgent, life-saving services, then pass the patient on to the specialist for long-term care and restoration to a healthy life.

The ED you use should be supervised twenty-four hours a day, seven days a week, by a team of emergency physicians (there are 2,000 or more of these specialists now, members of the American College of Emergency Physicians). Or else the ED should be in a university teaching hospital, where you are likely to find a somewhat different setup. In such a hospital the staff is so large and the back-up so extensive that it is possible to staff the ED adequately with residents (experienced interns, if you will) because there is always someone senior in the specialties available within minutes.

When you arrive in a community it's a simple matter to call the local hospitals, using the knowledge in our chapter on hospitals, and find out which have emergency physicians in charge of their EDs—or to locate the nearest university teaching hospital. Keep the address or location in mind, and the phone number handy.

Emergency physicians are often active in the initial training of EMTs and in their on-going education, and many make a point of working with these paraprofessionals in the ED. By giving twenty-four-hour coverage to the ED they are ideal for direct two-way radio ties with the ambulances that bring in the emergencies: this way the EMTs can get instructions on the care of their patients when the EKGs are transmitted or when they report in.

The results of a survey of EDs in the state of Washington (reported in the September 1973 *Bulletin of the American College of Surgeons*) are most revealing. The first comprehensive statewide survey of its kind, it found that hospitals connected with the University of Washington School of Medicine showed better physician coverage, equipment, and utilization than the other EDs: further proof of the value of a university teaching hospital. In the EDs, too, physician excellence was directly related to hospital size. The survey also found increasing utilization of emergency physicians on a full-time basis.

So this part of the problem is relatively simple: call the local hospitals and ask whether their EDs are staffed by emergency physicians who are members of the American College of Emergency Physicians; or locate a nearby university teaching hospital. In either case you stand a good chance of getting the best emergency medical care available. And you might well question moving into any community where such protection is not readily available.

Accidental Poisoning

This can happen to both adults and children, but children are the chief victims—nearly 2 million of them are poisoned every year, and their deaths run into the thousands (these figures are considered by some to be only the tip of the iceberg). There are precautions you can take to prevent this—and steps you *must* take if it happens.

Toddlers and pre-school children are the victims nine times out of ten. Many of the hundreds of thousands of household products contain chemicals poisonous to a child, but half of all poisonings are due to: aspirin (the worst offender and greatest killer); insecticides; household bleach; soaps, detergents, and cleaners; furniture polishes; kerosene; vitamin and iron compounds; deodorizers and disinfectants; laxatives; corrosives and lye. However, this list can change overnight with the introduction of a popular new household product or drug (the Pill and methadone are typical).

Preventing Poisoning:
The Danger Times and Situations

A recent investigation, at the famed Karolinska Institute in Stockholm, Sweden, helps to alert parents to certain dangers. This study of 600 childhood victims of accidental poisoning showed that no social or economic group is safe—and in 75 per cent of these incidents at least one parent was at home. Most poisonings occurred in the kitchen, usually during short periods when the child was alone. Moreover, these incidents peaked when the child was hungry, before meals—between 11 a.m. and noon, and 4 and 6 p.m. A brother or sister contributed to the accident in 2 per cent of the cases. While an older child may know enough not to take pills himself, he may still feed them to a small sister or brother.

It is well worth repeating some protective measures to prevent accidental poisoning. No potentially poisonous substance should ever be kept where a child can get a chair or place a box on a table and reach it—and medicine chests should *never* be used for drugs. Medication (even ordinary aspirin) should be locked away where the child can't possibly get at it. Also, never put poisonous products in a container that a child may associate with food or drink (a cup, glass, or soda bottle). This has repeatedly led to poisoning of adults as well as children. And don't depend on child-resistant containers—youngsters can easily use their teeth to remove a cap that an adult has difficulty in manipulating.

What to Do in Case of Accidental Poisoning

Always keep what is left (a few pills, the medicine bottle, or other container), for this identification may save a life by telling the experts what drug was involved so they can counteract it. With the bottle or container in your hand, telephone for advice *immediately*. If you can't reach your doctor, try the local Poison Control Center (it's wise to have this number in a convenient spot if you have small children); or call your local hospital (it's wise to have the phone number of the best hospital, too). If all else fails, call the police.

But whatever else—*don't delay,* and *always tell the truth about how much your child has taken.* One mother recently told the Duke University Poison Control Center that her child had taken three or four iron tablets—yet the medical people found thirty or forty tablets in the child. An untruth (sometimes because the distraught mother doesn't want the child put through stomach washing) can cost a child's life.

And, finally, it's wise to keep an ounce bottle of syrup of ipecac and a container of activated charcoal available—your doctor or poison expert may advise their use immediately, over the telephone.

The Breath of Life: CPR

Recently a middle-aged woman was hanging a picture and asked her son to hand her a hammer. When he turned with it she was dead—no heartbeat and no breathing. On a golf course, a man in his late fifties bent over to putt and suddenly pitched forward, also dead, with no heartbeat or breathing. Yet I met both of those people recently—for CPR had brought them back to life, and they now have every reason to look forward to a normal life expectancy. The same thing happened to a spectator at the 'Gator Bowl on New Year's Day in 1969, and to innumerable others. Dr. Roy M. Baker, Jacksonville's civic-minded and nationally known heart specialist, estimates conservatively that an average of two people a week have been brought back from death in his community, thanks to CPR.

It's not done with mirrors or by magic—in fact, the technique of CPR is so simple that experts say an eleven-year-old can be taught to use it, and Dr. Baker recalls instructing distraught wives how to do it by telephone in the small hours of the morning. In fact, Dr. Baker is helping to spearhead a drive to train every one of Jacksonville's citizens in CPR. Many other experts also feel this is the way to cut down our tragic toll of heart-attack deaths.

CPR—cardiopulmonary resuscitation—is literally putting the breath of life back into a person. A person who is "clinically dead," with no heartbeat and no breathing, can be brought back to life without damage if breathing and circulation are restored within four minutes. In CPR the rescuer becomes the victim's heart and lungs: by mouth-to-mouth breathing he supplies oxygen and by pressing on the breastbone he squeezes blood out of the heart and circulates it through the body. But there are only four minutes— longer than that without oxygen and the brain cells die; the person may still be revived but will end up as a vegetable.

Points to Remember

1. In the community where you live or visit, locate and record the phone numbers and addresses of the best local hospital emergency department and ambulance service; with small children,

also the nearest Poison Control Center. Get in the habit of doing this even if you're only visiting for a matter of days or weeks, and particularly if there are any health problems in your family.

2. Get the name of the best ambulance service from a doctor (an emergency physician if possible) in a good ED, or locate one yourself and check to be sure that at least two people (attendant and driver) ride the vehicle on each call, that both are EMTs or equivalents (sometimes volunteer services have people who qualify for EMT patches but just don't bother to take the necessary examinations).

3. Check the local hospitals to find the best ED. This will either be one staffed with emergency physicians (specialists and members of the American College of Emergency Physicians) on a full-time basis (24 hours a day, 7 days a week) or it will be in a university teaching hospital (the main hospital for a medical school).

4. Avoid accidental poisoning by keeping medications properly labeled and out of children's reach. Have an ounce bottle of syrup of ipecac and a container of activated charcoal on hand in case you are instructed by an expert to use them.

5. In case of accidental poisoning, make sure to keep any remaining pills or liquid and the bottle as well. With this in your hand, *immediately* call your doctor; if you can't reach him, try the nearest Poison Control Center, then the local hospital, in that order. If you still can't get help, call the police. Whomever you do reach, *always tell the full truth about what and how much your child has taken.*

6. Particularly if someone in your family has already had a heart attack, it's wise to learn CPR, but it's a good thing in any case—it's simple and it may save a life. Knowledge of advanced first aid is also of value.

Now we turn from the bodily medical ills to the emotional and psychological problems.

6

What You Must Know to Find the Right Psychiatrist

It's long been one of those things that pass for a joke in medical circles that it really doesn't matter if a psychiatrist is worthless or even an outright quack—since psychiatrists accomplish so little, there's really little danger of their doing any harm.

All this sounds very glib—only it's entirely false, of course. A psychiatrist, like any other physician or surgeon, can do a great deal of damage if he's incompetent or off base or just money-hungry. After all, the psychiatrist is tinkering with your mind, the very quality of life itself, and our emotions are so complex that we don't wish to risk having them scrambled up for us. Which is one reason why many observers feel it's usually safer to turn to psychiatrists for psychotherapy than to any of the other professionals now pouring into this field. But before we go into the types of help available, psychotherapy itself needs a bit of explaining.

What Is Psychotherapy and When Is It Needed?

Psychotherapy is, in more than one sense, virtually a modern form of faith healing. Actually, the term calls for an explanation rather than the simple cut-and-dried definition given in a dictionary, which is likely to be some variant of this line: *the treatment or curing of psychological and emotional, mental, and nervous disorders by psychological means.*

Psychotherapy is truly one of the healing arts (and it *is* an art, not a science). The patient is an unhappy person, suffering, distressed, perhaps even disabled by his emotional or psychological problems. Essentially, psychotherapy is a verbal treatment that seeks to influence the sufferer to change his behavior or his attitudes so that his suffering is relieved.

The suffering can be simple and obvious or manifold and complex, and can assume many forms. Take Myron. In his mid-thirties he suddenly changed from an active, successful business-man to a haunted, old-looking man no longer able to leave his home. All because one day, when he'd gone out, his strength drained away and his heart pounded wildly, while he panted in an effort to catch his breath. Certain he had had a heart attack, he became incapable of leaving his house without his wife. The few times he went to the neighborhood store he took a roundabout route so he'd have a wall he could cling to.

Sound unusual? Not really, for some 16 million Americans suffer from Myron's problem, and 500,000 of them are just as severely affected. This is what is really meant when experts talk of a "phobia." It keeps some people from flying, makes others become virtually disabled (women become "housebound housewives" and men give up their jobs). But these are not the only psychological problems, for Masters and Johnson estimate that at least half of our marriages either are sexually dysfunctional for psychological reasons or may well become so.

Take Wilma. Suffering headaches nearly all the time, she would sit up watching the *Late Late Show* on TV because she was unable to sleep. She felt no interest in sex, ate little, and during the day found it extremely difficult to take care of even the small apartment she and her husband lived in. She found life meaningless and took no pleasure in anything she did, would often break into tears without adequate reason, felt tired and worn despite her relative inactivity.

In short, Wilma was suffering from depression, a condition that has virtually become epidemic in the United States and is certainly our leading mental illness. In Scandinavia there are reports that 4 per cent of the population have this condition, while the famous Midtown Manhattan Study found 24 per cent suffering from it. It's been said that one in eight Americans will during his or her lifetime (it's about twice as common in women as in men) have a depression sufficiently severe to require psychotherapeutic help.

Myron and Wilma are only two of the many people who need psychotherapy. So do all of us with emotional problems bad enough to make us unhappy or cause us difficulties in handling our lives (producing divorces, recurrent problems in job or school or home, psychosomatic illnesses such as asthma, chronic headaches, stomach ulcers, or whatever).

The Kinds of Psychotherapy: Which Is Best?

There are many kinds of psychotherapy—from classical Freudian psychoanalysis, with its long-drawn-out individual therapy, to the latest short-term group or family therapy. There's behavior therapy and operant conditioning; there are therapists who follow the teachings of Jung or Adler or Reich; there are the new encounter groups and all sorts of way-out ideas and approaches.

The numbers of those who seek this help are amazingly large. According to the 1973 AMA statistics, there are some 20,000 psychiatrists involved in patient care (over 11,000 of them are office-based, the rest in hospitals), and psychiatrists had an average of 46.5 patient-visits each week in 1971. So just at a guess there must be several hundred thousand people who undergo therapy with psychiatrists every year, and the number who seek help from clinical psychologists and psychiatric social workers may be even larger.

Experts agree that decades of intensive study have failed to produce scientific proof that any one form of psychotherapy is more effective than any other in treating the majority of psychiatric problems. It's really a matter of matching the therapy to the patient, not trying to fit the patient into the straitjacket of any one particular therapy.

Dr. Jerome D. Frank, Johns Hopkins professor of psychiatry, regards psychotherapy as those procedures with three characteristics: where there is a "trained, socially sanctioned healer" whose curative powers are accepted by both the patient and his social group; where the patient or sufferer seeks help from this healer; and where there is a limited, organized series of meetings (appointments, for example) between healer and sufferer by means of which, often with the help of a group, the healer strives to change the patient's psychological condition or make-up, mainly by words and actions.

This characterization of psychotherapy would include such things as faith healing, religious conversion, the offbeat new therapies now being practiced, and even some of the tinkering with altered states of consciousness that one often hears about today. The proof of the value of any kind of psychotherapery is simple: if a therapy has managed to last, it must be doing some good or it would have disappeared. On the other hand, as Dr. Frank points out (in what amounts to a disproof of the joke with which we started this chapter), the very fact that psychotherapy does make some of its patients worse is proof of the power it really possesses. But what of the person who wields this powerful healing and helping tool, the psychotherapist?

Why a Psychiatrist
and Not Just Any Psychotherapist?

A variety of professionals, semi-professionals, and sub-professionals, and some just plain quacks have entered this field today. This has happened for a number of reasons, not the least, no doubt, being the fact that psychology and social work have captured the imagination of so many young people. Perhaps the increasing interest in the occult and in altered states of consciousness has also opened the way to this explosion. Another contributing factor is the laws governing therapists, which vary from state to state. Though most states require licensing or certification of those who want to call themselves "psychologists," anyone at all can bill himself as a "psychotherapist" or "marriage counselor." Many ministers are becoming involved in pastoral counseling, and psychiatric social workers too are doing psychotherapy.

It would seem the height of folly to entrust one's mental and emotional stability to a person who answers to no overseeing authority, whose qualifications you have no way of checking, whose basic abilities have not been tested in any way.

Typical of the mushrooming growth in these fields is the growth in numbers of psychologists. According to *Health Resources Statistics*, put out by the United States National Center for

Health Statistics, the number of psychologists engaged in health activities jumped from 3,000 in 1950 to nearly 9,000 in 1965; while the number with doctorates (usually Ph.D.s) went from 820 in 1960–61 to 2,116 in 1970–71. But of the 27,000 psychologists in the June 1973 issue of *Health Resources Statistics,* there were only 1,191 in private practice.

Psychologists get their training not in separate professional schools (such as medical schools) but in the graduate departments of psychology of some 150 universities that offer doctoral programs. They are often denied opportunities for psychoanalytic training in the United States because to do psychoanalysis a medical degree is required. This is no reflection on the individual clinical psychologist, who is often more research-oriented than the psychiatrist (and many psychologists have become leading psychotherapists). But it does make it impossible to judge psychologists as objectively as one can psychiatrists. Moreover, since there are some 12,000 psychiatrists in private practice, you are, by the very weight of numbers, ten times as likely to seek therapy with a psychiatrist as with a psychologist. For all these reasons, this chapter has been limited to ways of choosing a psychiatrist (although many of the ways we will discuss can be applied to clinical psychologists as well).

There are other reasons why psychiatrists are considered preferable by many observers of the psychotherapy scene. Since the psychiatrist has a medical background, he should be more capable of identifying the physical problem that may underly the emotional. He should be more capable of discovering when psychosomatic disorders are present and pointing out the medical realities of any illness. If a patient complains of physical symptoms in the course of therapy, the psychiatrist should recognize whether these symptoms are even possible given the case (certain pains have nothing to do with cancer, for example).

Finally, the psychiatrist is a licensed physician. This acts as a check on irresponsibility, for, in extreme cases, he does have a license to lose. Moreover, the possibility of complaints to his specialty organizations (he should have his boards in neurology and psychiatry and be a member of the American Psychiatric Association) is a threat to a practitioner who is not carrying out his duties conscientiously and ethically.

Is This Psychiatrist Right for You?

With psychiatrists, more than with any other physician, only a personal meeting can verify a good doctor-patient "fit." You may well have to do a good deal of shopping (couch-hopping, if you will) before you actually find the right one for you. You may not like your surgeon; you and your ophthalmologist may not hit it off at all; you may feel your dermatologist is interested only in that one tiny patch of skin and couldn't care less about you and your feelings. Yet you may still seek these men's or women's medical help, recognizing that they are competent professionals in a distinctly limited area and that you can use them to resolve your particular medical problem.

In psychiatry any such feelings would absolutely disqualify the specialist from helping you. In fact, even the psychiatrist who helped your wife or best friend or brother may not be able to help you, simply because you two don't hit it off. If that strange interrelationship which springs up between two people, even if they only say "Hi" once in a while, is not just right, then the finest psychiatrist in the world won't be able to help *you*.

With your psychiatrist, more than with any other physician, your feeling about him must be right. You have to like him (or her) and feel comfortable with him, and he must feel the same about you. The psychiatrist too has his likes and dislikes, hang-ups, strengths, and weaknesses. None of us ever lives long enough to eliminate every last psychological quirk.

You've no doubt heard of a psychiatrist who uses psychoanalysis, or of another who's using the newer behavior therapy; then there are those who work with group or family therapy. Today there are more techniques than you can count, each with its followers who swear by it. Many leading experts feel there's a strong likelihood that it is neither the method nor the technique that really determines success, but the magic doctor-patient relationship so vital in all medical practice. In psychotherapy this relationship becomes the most powerful of all medicines.

Clearly, in psychiatry it's absolutely essential to find a practitioner to whom you can relate well, with whom you're comfortable—or you're not likely to get very much help. If the relationship is not good, it is no reflection on either you or the psychiatrist. It just means that somewhere in your unconscious mind something has prevented the necessary rapport. When this happens—and it's not uncommon—you're much better off saying, "Thank you, Doctor," and looking for another office where the feeling is right for you.

If this should happen time after time, then you must consider the possibility that the problem really lies within you. It might be time to light somewhere and fight out the problem with the best psychiatrist you can find.

How Do You Find a Psychiatrist?

This is a particularly tricky area because of the emotional reaction so many people—physicians and laymen alike—still have to psychiatry. To begin, you can stay away from referrals by friends or business people, and follow the other suggestions offered in the chapter on finding a family doctor. If you've succeeded in obtaining a good family physician, he's certainly the best one to ask, unless he has something against psychiatry.

A referral from your family doctor—or any physician, for that matter—is usually safe, but you might also ask the referring doctor, "Have you referred patients to him before?" And if the answer is "yes," then ask, "How successful was he in helping them?" You might also ask, "Has he helped patients with problems like mine?" As in any other field, some psychiatrists are more successful in handling certain types of difficulties than others. If you can contact a nurse in the psychiatric service of a hospital or serving in a psychiatric hospital, you may learn some valuable information about the psychiatrists with whom she works—how concerned they are with their patients and how successful, what their colleagues think of them.

If all these approaches draw a blank, you can fall back on a call to the local medical school or the university teaching hospital or even the largest community hospital: you can get a list of those available for private patients or you might simply ask for the chief of psychiatry. So much depends on the interaction between you and this doctor that these can only be vague guidelines and tell little about how good he'll be for *you*.

What You Should Look For in a Psychiatrist

• First, of course, he should be board-certified in both neurology and psychiatry. If he's on the staff of a medical school or a hospital, find out what rank he has.

• Don't be surprised if, when you call a psychiatrist you get an answering service that takes only your name and phone number. Many (if not most) psychiatrists don't have secretaries and call you back personally later in the day, probably between patients.

• The psychiatrist, or psychotherapist, should be mature with broad personal experience. As one leading East Coast therapist told me, "I knew all the terms and theories before I was forty-five years old, but, looking back, I now realize that I really couldn't practice properly before my mid-forties. You just haven't lived long enough." A midwestern professor of psychiatry put it this way: "You need a therapist who's had at least twenty years of experience behind him." Age and experience can be determined either by asking your psychiatrist or by checking in the library, as you did with your family doctor.

• You should find the psychiatrist a decent human being—sincere, warm, non-critical, and responsive in an emergency. (One New York psychiatrist surprised his patient Alan by spending an hour on the telephone with him—Alan needed help but the psychiatrist couldn't see him that day at his office because of hospital commitments.) Many psychiatrists deliberately make themselves available at home by phone for emergencies.

• Your psychiatrist should be conversant with what's going on in the world around him and be able to relate to your job and your career no matter what it is. He should be clearly at ease with your life-style—or you need another therapist.

• Certainly the psychiatrist who makes sexual advances to a patient is one to avoid, despite the growing numbers of such reports.

• You should be able to ask your therapist if he's undergone analysis himself (if he hasn't, he may still have hang-ups that will make him unable to give you the help *you* need).

• Ask your therapist about the type of therapy he utilizes. If he seems too enthusiastic about using only one approach, he's wrong for you. A therapist must be broad-based and flexible, recognizing that no one therapeutic approach suits every patient. He should be prepared to refer you to another psychiatrist if you need a technique he's not comfortable with.

• Ask how successful your therapist has been with *your* type of problems. If he tells you he's never succeeded with them, you know you'd better get another psychiatrist.

• You should feel perfectly comfortable in telling your therapist anything, in saying anything in any way you feel like. This is an absolute essential.

Your Job in Psychiatry

Your psychiatrist is not God; he can't read what's going on in your mind. You have to tell him what you feel; if you don't, you're only cheating yourself, and you can't blame him for any failures. On the other hand, he should be prepared and able to admit when he's wrong. For instance, Alice accused her psychiatrist of not paying attention to her on one visit. He apologized and admitted he'd been up all night with his sick child and his attention had lagged. If he had denied his inattention, it would have damaged their relationship.

The psychiatrist must also be able to share his feeling with you. When Charles learned his psychiatrist's wife had died, he brought up the subject. The psychiatrist told Charles how he felt, then added, "How could I expect my patients to respect what I say to them when they suffer a loss if I can't do it myself, if I'm not prepared to be open and honest about myself?"

You have to like and respect your psychiatrist, and he must feel the same about you, but you have no more right to expect him to be perfect than he will expect it of you. You are both human beings, sharing problems and experiences together. In short, he should be the sort of person you would want to know even if he weren't your psychiatrist.

You do have one specific responsibility when dealing with psychiatrists: you must be exactly on time. These physicians work by a very precise time schedule. If your appointment is for 9:25, he will be ready for you at 9:25—at least four times out of five (the fifth time won't be his fault, and even then he won't be more than a few minutes late). If you are late, your appointment will end at its regular time, and so you will only cheat yourself of the time you pay for.

Psychotherapy is feared simply because it means facing up to the truth about yourself, looking at the deep feelings you're trying to conceal. There is probably only one other professional who is as much feared as the psychiatrist, and that is the one we will discuss in our next chapter—the dentist.

7

How to Find and Use a Dentist--
without Being Used

Dentistry involves every one of us. Even if we never have a cavity we still need our teeth cleaned and checked regularly. According to recent estimates, there are almost a billion unfilled cavities in American teeth, more than four for every man, woman, and child in the country. Some $4 billion a year is spent for dental care, according to the American Dental Association (ADA)—and that kind of money is certainly an attraction to the unscrupulous or fraudulent, the inadequate or incompetent, or the just plain dishonest dentist.

Add to all this the intense American desire for youth and perfection, the great fear of pain, and the desire to avoid any semblance of artificial replacements and you have powerful temptations to those who want to practice unnecessary dentistry. This poses a threat to your pocketbook as well as your health, because dental bills can run into thousands of dollars, and some of the new experimental techniques are extensive as well as expensive.

Dentistry as a profession is very young compared to medicine —the first American dental school was established just before the Civil War. And dentistry is distinctly behind medicine as a healing profession. There is less research, and there is less recognition of professional involvement. The physician who takes the trouble to write a medical book or article for a professional journal is quickly recognized, whereas the dentist who does this is not. Few dentists turn to specialized work or utilize specialists; few are on hospital staffs or take internships or residencies.

In general, dentistry is a more mechanical profession than medicine, except for some medical specialties. The dentist is far more likely to be concerned with the mechanics and looks of his special area than with the total patient. The dentist is also more likely to be striving for status. If you want to handle him well, don't ever speak to him of "doctors and dentists," or you will have an enemy instead of an ally, for he treasures being considered a "doctor" too.

What Protection Do You Have from the Dishonest or Unqualified Dentist?

Virtually only your own ability to check what he's doing! Dr. Denenberg, whose interest in the consumer has been mentioned earlier, recently published "A Shopper's Guide to Dentistry," which is well worth obtaining. In it he points out that Pennsylvania (like nearly all states) does not have the manpower, the resources, or the laws to protect its citizens against the unqualified, incompetent, or dishonest dentist—any more than it can protect against the irresponsible physician. In a period of five years, through 1972, only one Pennsylvania dentist lost his license.

Nor can you expect any protection from the dental societies at any level—national, state, county, or local. Dr. Denenberg reports a letter from the Pennsylvania Dental Association indicating that it had disciplined *no* dentists—nor had the local societies, to the best of the state association's knowledge. And certainly no other state is likely to show a better record.

As with physicians, conservative estimates show that at least 15 per cent of dentists are unqualified, incompetent, or dishonest —and these figures are considered far, far too low by many. Some even talk in terms of half the dental practitioners! And when you realize that the National Center for Health Statistics found that in 1971 there were 311,943,000 visits made to dentists, that 92 million of these visits were for fillings and 38 million for extractions and other surgery, you can begin to get a feeling for the seriousness of incompetence in this field.

How Good Is Dentistry in General?

Not good—which is why you have to learn to protect yourself. Sincere, competent practitioners invariably are shocked at the poor level of general dental care, and figures now available substantiate this. Dr. Denenberg calls attention to a check made on the dentistry done for 1,300 Medicaid patients in New York State: 9 per cent was inexcusably bad, while another 9 per cent was outright fraudulent. The accuracy of these figures is difficult to judge, since only 1,300 patients made themselves available for the check-up, out of the 6,000 asked to come in. Other figures indicate that 25 per cent of all the New York Medicaid dental treatment was unnecessary. A later, much larger, sample of patients—some 11,000—revealed that only four out of five (some 81.2 per cent) patients got satisfactory dentistry. A recent ADA survey found that only one dentist in four used a lead apron to protect his patients from dental x-rays, which should always be done.

Why Is Dentistry So Inadequate?

Dentistry is still a "cottage industry." As of 1968, seven out of ten dentists practiced entirely alone in their offices, while most of the rest merely shared the physical setup of their offices with another dentist, without any professional connections. Only one dentist in twenty actually was a part of a group practice, a situation in which there would be an opportunity to see what the other practitioners were doing and thus in some measure provide a sort of peer review.

To make matters worse, the dental student's motivations are clearly expressed in what one young college student told me: "I want to become a dentist because it's a nice clean way of making a good living and people look up to you." Scientific studies have shown that desires for financial rewards and prestige motivate the dental student right from the beginning. A highly cynical attitude appears in 10 per cent of the freshman class and increases to affect nearly one-third of the seniors; while the high ideals present in about two-thirds of the entering students were found in barely a quarter of the seniors.

This cottage-industry character of dentistry has resulted from its total self-containment and its independence from any outside resources, such as the hospital, skilled technicians in medical and x-ray laboratories, most specialists, or complex treatment facilities. The result is that the dentist's work is rarely—and then almost only by accident—seen by other professionals qualified to judge it. Lack of scrutiny by other professionals invariably removes an important and necessary motivating force in good practice.

Our health-care system imposes serious limitations on the dental practitioners. Only very rarely does a dentist have any real need for a hospital affiliation, and so he has little if any contact with other dentists except in the dental societies, which are very limited as a means of providing professional training. Only a miniscule proportion of dentists ever carry out their procedures in the view of another dentist (a surgeon, in contrast, performs in the presence of an anesthesiologist, assistants, and operating-room nurses).

Reducing the opportunities to share professional experiences even further, probably at most one in ten dentists actually joins in continuing education each year. In addition, the dental profession has suffered from a problem just the opposite of the medical profession's. Whereas the physicians have seen an increasing fragmentation of their profession into specialties, dentistry has failed to adequately develop and utilize its specialties. To ensure proper dentistry, you had better learn what specialties are available to you.

The Specialties of Dentistry

There are eight dental specialties in which boards (comparable to those in medicine) are available. But of some 123,000 dentists in the United States in 1972, fewer than one in ten (a little over 11,000) is a specialist.

The oldest, largest, and by far the most familiar specialty is orthodontics. In 1972 there were slightly over 4,500 orthodontists in the United States. In general, orthodontistry is the most complete of the dental specialties. Relatively few general dental practitioners venture into it, perhaps because dental schools provide the generalist only a limited training in the field.

Second only to orthodontics in length of existence, size, and familiarity to the public is oral surgery, with just over 2,700 practitioners in 1972. It is an underused specialty, for general dental practitioners probably still do at least half the surgical procedures—everything from simple extractions to the complicated removal of impacted wisdom teeth. Some have even been known to get involved in the removal of soft-tissue conditions that eventually proved to be malignant growths.

This intrusion of the general dental practitioner into the practice of dental specialties and the generally inadequate utilization of these specialties are more evidence of the fact that dentistry is still considerably behind medicine (at least twenty-five years, and perhaps fifty). In fact, there are only two specialties that the general dental practitioner doesn't dominate in terms of actual amounts of work done and numbers of patients treated.

Pedodontics and periodontics are almost in a tie for third place in familiarity to the public, length of existence, and size, with a little over 1,200 pedodontists and 1,100 periodontists in 1972.

Pedodontics is the specialty which, like pediatrics, deals with the care of children; but the "children" cared for by the pedodontist range up to fifteen or sixteen years of age. This is simply because the pedodontist can't get enough five- or six-year-olds to make a living, for the increasing fluoridation of water has produced a marked decrease in cavities among young children. This effect has been most noticeable in areas such as Maryland, the District of Columbia, and Virginia, where the drinking water has been heavily fluoridated.

Periodontics is the care and treatment of diseases of the gums and bones that support the teeth. These disorders, formerly called "pyorrhea" and now termed "periodontal disease," will eventually lead to loosening of the teeth if untreated (and sometimes even when treated).

Prosthodontics (it used to be called "prosthetics") is fifth among the dental specialties in its length of existence, familiarity to the public, and size (700 prosthodontists in 1972). The prosthodontist is the dental equivalent of the internist in medicine, for he usually practices general dentistry in addition to his specialty, which is the making of dentures (full dentures are what were once called "plates"), bridges, crowns, and other complex replacements and restorations. The line between prosthodontics and general dentistry is a fine one indeed, except that the prosthodontist is board-certified and presumably has a greater knowledge of his specialty, sometimes called "rehabilitation." However, the bulk of prosthodontics is probably performed by general practitioners.

Endodontics is sixth among the dental specialties and well down the line in length of existence, familiarity to the public, and size (fewer than 600 endodontists in 1972). These are the dentists who specialize in "root canal therapy" (devitalizing teeth) and deal with the nerves of the teeth. In general, their job is to save abscessed and "dead" teeth. Many will perform surgery called "apicoectomy," or root-end amputation. Cutting through gum and bone, they remove a cyst or abscess at the end of the root to save the tooth. The great bulk of endodontics is done by general practitioners.

The last two specialties are relatively minor in the spectrum of dental practice. Oral pathology is the study of diseases of the tissues of the mouth, their diagnosis and treatment. This may include bone conditions of many sorts in the jaws, diseases of the soft tissues (gums, cheeks, lips, palatal tissues, tongue, and so on). Oral pathologists perform biopsies and study tissues under the microscope in order to diagnose the infection, tumor, or whatever. It is a recent specialty and barely known to the public; there were only 120 oral pathologists in 1972.

Eighth and newest of the dental specialties is dental public health, with 116 such specialists in 1972. These are the people concerned with the overview, dental care for the community as a whole as opposed to the individual patient. They study, for example, dental care and education in the schools, fluoridation of the water supply, and dental care for the needy, and form the dental sections of the various governmental public health departments.

How to Select a Specialist
or a General Practitioner

All dentists have one of two degrees: D.D.S. (doctor of dental surgery) or D.M.D. (doctor of dental medicine), and these are exactly alike. The two terms have arisen because different schools (teaching exactly the same things) have historically given these different degrees. Remember that surgery is the treatment of disease by manipulation (which is what the dentist does when he drills your teeth and fills them), whereas medicine is the treatment of disease by drugs (which a dentist may do by giving an antibiotic for an infection). So if you see "Dental Surgeon" on a shingle it means only that this man is a dentist, nothing more. Extractions, removals of impacted teeth, and other operations are traditionally called "oral surgery," so an "oral surgeon" is a dentist who performs the true surgery of the mouth. A bit confusing, but long usage has made it this way.

The oral surgeon or any other dental specialist you use should be board-certified, just as medical specialists are. But the qualifications of the general dental practitioner are difficult to judge. Your family dentist will not be board-certified, as is the F.P. or the internist. Still, you can look for the school the dentist was graduated from—American dental schools are still the best, and their quality is roughly equivalent to that of the university to which they are attached (Harvard, Michigan, or California, or whatever).

Certainly the proof of any dental work is in how well it stands up to time and usage. If the fillings fall out each time you eat, if the teeth loosen up without warning after years of regular care by the same dentist, if teeth develop abscesses, if bridges don't function adequately—you've got the wrong person. But besides trial and error, there are other things you can check.

How to Tell if a Dentist Is Qualified

When you're considering a new dentist, you can start by checking his qualifications. Does he teach in a dental school? Is he on the staff of a really good hospital? A "yes" answer to one of these at least indicates that the dentist is exposed to the newest techniques. The dental societies do a lot of post-graduate teaching, and a dentist who teaches or lectures for one of these is also likely to be up to date.

In the last analysis, though, only the test of time is meaningful. Some of the best dentists I've known are independent of any professional affiliations, and some of the poorest are professors. But, in general, you're safer with someone who does teach. Also, try to find out how much time he devotes—if any—to his own continuing education in the form of post-graduate courses, lectures, reading dental journals, and so on.

Membership in the ADA (and thus automatically in the local dental association) means only that some lectures and courses are available to the dentist; there are no requirements for attending meetings or keeping up with the times. Becoming a member is easy and really indicates only that he hasn't been involved in gross problems—specifically, he hasn't clashed with fellow practitioners in ways that are considered "unethical," which essentially means he hasn't said anything negative to a patient about another dentist's work or about the profession. In short, you'll get no more protection from the ADA than from the AMA.

Finding a Family Dentist

Just as with physicians, the good dental generalist is harder to find than the specialist. It may well entail many false starts and any number of changes, but your health, your teeth, and your pocket all deserve the effort. Remember that half or more of dentistry may well be inadequate, incompetent, or downright unnecessary. But, unlike medicine, it's harder to pin down objective qualifications, and there are fewer ways to find an adequate practitioner.

Probably an ideal way to get a family dentist is by referral from another practitioner who has seen his work and is qualified to judge it. If you have a good friend who is an orthodontist, an oral surgeon, a periodontist, or endodontist (a prosthodontist is probably doing general dentistry himself), he would be in an ideal position to see the work done by a general practitioner and judge its over-all quality. I emphasize "good friend" because otherwise the specialist may be referring you as a way of paying back a dentist who sends him referrals, a form of ethical fee-splitting, as it were.

Another useful source is a dental hygienist who has worked with a number of dentists or in an office where she sees the work of a range of men—but this depends in part on her expertise and how much attention she pays to dentistry as well as to her own work of cleaning teeth. Physicians are usually not particularly good sources of referral, because they are more impressed with the medical knowledge of the dentist and not sufficiently familiar with the technical aspects of dentistry.

As a last resort you can ask someone who's been treated by a dentist for a considerable number of years and can tell from experience how his work stands up.

What to Look for in Your Dentist

The worst test you can use is how busy the practitioner is. For one thing, good dentists run their practices on very strict appointment schedules and you'll rarely find anybody else sitting in the reception room while you're there. In fact, if you arrive on time you should be shown into an office almost immediately, and ideally you should be dismissed a few moments before the next patient arrives. A strict appointment schedule with only one person waiting when you leave is evidence that the dentist respects your time as well as his own. There are some dentists who deliberately jam all their appointments into a few hours of certain days so that they always seem busy, even though they may not have enough patients to fill a normal week.

The first appointment should include a careful medical and dental history—to protect you. This can prevent serious damage being done to "bleeders" or to people with certain heart conditions or allergies. You should also test the dentist's approach to specialization, as you did the physician's. Ask to whom he refers his extractions, and if he says he'll always try to save your tooth but if necessary he uses Dr. X, it's a good sign. It's easier to check an oral surgeon, for he should have a hospital appointment or teaching position.

Then you can ask how the dentist handles root-canal therapy. Many practitioners do single-rooted teeth themselves but should be prepared to refer multi-rooted teeth to specialists. And you might ask if there's any particular area of dentistry he's particularly interested in—this may lead him on to tell you something of his post-graduate study and how seriously he takes his work. Once he starts talking of his interest he may go on to tell you of specialty societies and the meetings he attends regularly—an indication of how active and up to date he is.

If the dentist starts talking of complicated work, you might ask him what specialized training he's had in it—and if he becomes defensive you have a warning. He should be quite open about his basic training and what he's done to keep it up to date, what he does with special problems, and how he feels about consultation for extensive work. All this will give you a feel for the man and his practice of dentistry.

The First Examination

We have already mentioned the medical and dental history. The first examination should also include x-rays, unless you've had them within the last year or two. If these are good ones, the new dentist should not re-expose you—and his use of x-rays is another check. He should be concerned with protecting you from radiation by always using a lead apron, by using ultra-fast x-ray film, and by underexposing and overdeveloping it. Small, weak, foreign x-ray machines also add protection. A full-mouth x-ray series showing the roots of the teeth should be done only every one to two years, preferably two if there is no specific problem. "Bite-wings"—four or six—can be done every six months to a year, depending on your susceptibility to decay, with careful clinical examinations substituting whenever possible.

Question the dentist about his use of x-rays (they are definitely being overused) and his procedures. If he hedges, sneak a look at the back of the tiny x-rays. There you'll find the brand name and type, and you can check with your local health department on x-ray safety to be sure he's using the fast film they recommend. If he's careless about x-ray safety or gets a stiff back when you question him, you can be suspicious about other measures being taken to protect you.

The dentist should carefully examine the soft tissues of your mouth—the cheeks, lips, tongue, and floor of the mouth. He should look down your throat and under your tongue and on your palate —every place he can possibly see tissue. It's all part of the campaign against cancer—and it is his responsibility to do it. He may want impressions to show how your upper and lower teeth meet, as a long-term record. All of this indicates careful dentistry.

How to Discuss Needed Dental Work

If anything more than a cleaning and a filling or two is involved, ask to discuss the work in detail. Have the dentist show you on your x-rays the location of the cavities. It's easy to read dental x-rays, and competent dentists are always glad to have material available which illustrates their work. The ADA puts out a lot of useful material along these lines. You can go over your x-rays with the dentist and see whether what he says fits in with what you see. Use a hand mirror and ask to see the cavities. An old dental trick is to fill the groove on a tooth's biting surface in two or three spots instead of placing a single filling all along the indentation. You can't trust any dentist who would suggest several such pit fillings instead of a single large one.

Ask for details—and a written plan if any extensive work is recommended. Find out what types of fillings or bridges or other work he proposes. Make careful notes unless he will give you a written plan. Ask what other ways of doing the work there are, how complicated each procedure is and how long it will take, what each entails (how much cutting of tooth structure, what kind of temporary appliances will be available). Finally, discuss the various fees. If the dentist gets his back up at specific questions or refuses to detail precisely his recommendations and alternatives, be suspicious.

If the work is extensive or complex—"capping" or "rehabilitation," for example—ask if he would mind a consultation with a specialist. If he sees you are doubtful, a serious practitioner will urge a consultation and might suggest a list of three or more men you might choose from. Actually, it would be better for you to find your own expert. Take your x-rays and study models to him just for a consultation if you like the general practitioner you started with but want to check on him. Once you're sure, you may never need to check on him again, but it's good to do it the first time a lot of work looms up. If you're not sure about the practitioner, see another general practitioner with the thought of his doing the work; but if there's a lot of work to be done, always visit someone (a professor in that specialty is good) just for a consultation, with the frank statement that you have your dentist but want to find out what the specialist advises.

One important question is whether the work advised is an accepted or standard treatment. A good deal of highly experimental and controversial work (such as implants) is being done widely today. Before you even consider an experimental procedure, get a consultation with a professor of prosthodontics in a dental school if possible. Since this work can endanger your health and run into several thousand dollars, it certainly warrants one or two consultations before embarking on it.

Never hesitate to check one specialist with another. Dr. Denenberg even urges that you have a consultation before letting anyone extract a single tooth—which sounds extreme, except that the statistics on teeth lost unnecessarily bear out his suspicions.

A good family dentist is a person to treasure if you're lucky enough to find one!

Points to Remember

1. A good recommendation for a dentist is a patient who's satisfied with the dental work after many years.

2. Learn the dental specialties so you can ask for a referral or for a consultation when you need one.

3. Insist on a lead apron and fewer x-rays, fast films underexposed and overdeveloped, and learn to read them with your dentist (it's easy and in dentistry you have to protect yourself).

4. If there is considerable work to be done, ask for a detailed written breakdown (teeth involved, type of work, alternatives, fees, and so on). *Get a consultation*—don't go into extensive work (capping, rehabilitation, implants) without confirmation that you need it and that the work is *not* controversial or experimental.

PART II
Special Problems in Managing Your Doctors: How to Keep Yourself Safe from Medical Mayhem

8

Protecting Yourself against X-rays

Before you brush off the problem of x-rays as not applying to you, remember that in just the period of April through September 1970, the National Center for Health Statistics found 180 million visits made for x-rays in the United States (112 million of these for medical reasons and the rest dental). From 1964 to 1970 the number of individual Americans exposed to medical and dental x-rays increased from 108 million to 130 million—in short, roughly seven out of ten of us had x-rays taken and so were exposed to radiation to some extent.

Before you dismiss the subject with an "Oh well, an x-ray is nothing," remember that some experts have estimated—pessimistically perhaps but with a very real basis for concern—that thousands of cancers and leukemias are caused by x-rays, and that these diseases take some 3,500 to 30,000 lives a year. The promiscuous use of x-rays has become a disturbing element in the United States health-care system—a problem not only of unnecessary x-rays, but also of inadequate or untrained personnel, failure to protect the patient, and bad legal and insurance setups. The result: another health menace to *you,* the consumer, and especially if you are the kind of patient who ordinarily goes along with your doctor's advice. Perhaps the time has come to revolt, to speak out, to demand more personal care for *you.*

The facts are disturbing, to say the least. New York University found an increased incidence of cancer and mental illness in one sample of 2,000 patients treated with x-rays for ringworm of the scalp. X-rays are like cars—primarily safe and valuable tools in the hands of the competent and conscientious operator, but lethal weapons in the hands of the irresponsible, inadequate, or badly trained technician. A host of people (hospital committees, the Joint Commission on Accreditation, colleagues, and others) are constantly peering over the shoulders of the radiologists (doctors who specialize in x-rays) in the hospitals, and the quality of their work is likely to correspond to the quality of the hospital. But no one checks on the individual doctor who may have the $8,000 or $9,000 with which to buy a used x-ray machine, or who may even just rent one.

The results of the use of x-rays by non-radiologists are tragic. The chief of surgery at a major Pacific Coast hospital, writing under a pseudonym in the much respected medical magazine, *Medical Economics* October 1972, reported the case of a family physician who told his patient her gastro-intestinal x-rays showed nothing wrong. Three months later the films were checked by a specialist, who spotted a stomach cancer. Earlier surgery might have saved her life. In other incidents, a woman in her twenties was thrown into menopause by an overdose of x-rays; another woman was electrocuted; and a man lost both legs when treated with x-rays for eczema.

These may sound like isolated cases, but they're not. Radiologists are shocked by the way x-rays are thrown about. Non-radiologists—who take more x-rays than professional radiologists—can take the simpler films, but they can't really diagnose them. Repeatedly I've heard specialists comment, as one did about a specific G.P.: "He thinks he knows what he's doing but he just doesn't know what he's looking at."

Dr. John Knowles, now president of the Rockefeller Foundation but formerly in practice, had specialized training in radiology. He would often take the films of his patients himself, but after he'd read them he would turn them over to a radiologist to double-check that he hadn't missed anything. It's not taking the x-ray that's the problem—anybody can be taught that—but the interpretation, diagnosis, and evaluation of those vague and elusive shadows, those shades of gray or black, those irregular profiles and shapes and sizes. Reading an x-ray is truly an art, one that must constantly be practiced and studied to sharpen the expertise and to keep up to date with the rapidly changing practices in this field.

The radiologist rarely, if ever, takes x-rays himself. In any setup where a large number of x-rays are taken, you'll find technicians doing the actual work. In the major centers or the specialist's office, you're protected by adequately trained technicians, for radiologists know the needed qualifications and can judge them. But in only three states (New York, New Jersey, and California) and in Puerto Rico are radiologic technicians required to be licensed. Elsewhere x-rays may be taken by anybody taught to aim a machine.

Training x-ray personnel is a serious problem for the operators as well as the patients. One hospital technician, who did radiology for four years with no monitoring of his exposure, died of leukemia; another, who helped out in the x-ray room, holding patients who couldn't support themselves, suffered skin burns and anemia. Radiation is a double-edged sword that can strike both patient and operator when adequately trained personnel—radiologist or physician or technician—are not utilized.

What Has Caused the X-ray Problem?

This is a complex matter of money, insurance, law, emotion, and routine. First for the financial aspects: the G.P. who has bought an x-ray machine—perhaps investing $20,000 to $35,000 in a new one—is likely to want to "make it pay for itself." Not uncommon in American society in general, this attitude becomes dangerous when applied to health care, particularly when the physician or dentist either is not familiar with the hazards of x-rays or doesn't know how to interpret them.

Money is also part of the doctor's concern over malpractice suits, with their potential for notoriety, resultant loss of practice, and possibly increased insurance premiums. Because of their exaggerated fear of malpractice suits, physicians in general today tend to practice the so-called defensive medicine, ordering unnecessary tests and other procedures (such as x-rays) to be carried out only in order to protect themselves against such suits.

Insurance, too, contributes to the problem, in that it often pays for x-rays. This may lead physicians to overprescribe them, and the patient, who doesn't have to pay, usually does not object. Now there is even a pre-employment x-ray examination of the lower back being used in the belief that it can indicate the likelihood of future job-related lower-back problems—even though there is considerable evidence that this just isn't so.

The law too exacts its price. As Dr. John L. McClenahan, a professor of radiology at Philadelphia's Jefferson Medical College, points out in a much-quoted editorial in the medical journal *Radiology*, there are severe legal penalties for the doctor who doesn't get an x-ray regardless of the trifling nature of the injury or illness in question—but no penalty for unnecessary x-rays regardless of how many times repeated or how meaningless. It's been estimated that up to one-fifth of all x-rays are taken for medico-legal reasons. Of fifty-five skull x-rays in one study, only one showed anything wrong, according to Dr. Alexander R. Margulis, chairman of the Department of Radiology at the University of California Medical School, at San Francisco. Another study has shown that one-fifth of skull x-rays are done for very minor injuries, and more than a third only for medico-legal reasons.

Dr. McClenahan is frank in pointing out that x-rays are widely used not to diagnose injury but to treat the anxieties of either patient or doctor. He recalls how, in a three-year period, a thirteen-year-old boy underwent more than seventy-six x-rays of his spine, which had a congenital defect causing no problems or threats to his life. The surgeon was anxious about the viability of a corrective operation and wanted reassurance: yet at his patient's age a human being is most susceptible to x-ray damage, which can produce defects in his children.

Any radiologist's files are filled with thick envelopes of x-rays of people whose complaints and unhappy symptoms arose not from physical damage or medical conditions but from psychosomatic disorders. And innumerable x-rays are taken when a simple physical examination could establish the diagnosis accurately and with ease.

Then too there are the "routine" x-rays—as when Dave recently visited an internist in his search for a family doctor. A professor of medicine at a large East Coast medical school, Dave's internist, after a cursory physical examination, ordered x-rays of hand and thumb, hip, gall bladder, chest, and head, because Dave (in his mid-fifties) complained of some thumb and hip pain and gave a history of a gall-bladder attack and a brain abscess some fifteen years earlier. The internist wanted to check the cause of the thumb and hip pain (a clinical examination was all a specialist needed to recognize osteoarthritis); the head x-rays were "for the record" (no one else saw any specific reason for them); the gallbladder x-rays were "to see" (earlier x-rays had revealed nothing and no time was spent on consideration of this problem on its merits); and the chest x-rays were "routine." No real effort was made to think about any of these x-rays ordered on Dave—they were virtually all ordered "for the record," "routinely," "to see." To make matters worse, Dave was never seen by the private radiologist. A technician took his physician's order and ran the x-rays through, so Dave never even got a chance to question the radiologist as to their need—which was, to say the least, questionable.

Only recently has the use of "routine" x-rays for mass screening been condemned by the Food and Drug Administration, the American College of Chest Physicians, and the American College of Radiology. In fact, leading radiologists urge the individual consideration of every "routine" x-ray to reduce unnecessary radiation with all its attendant dangers. There are endless repetitions of x-rays "to be sure," or because the original x-rays can't be located immediately, or for other invalid reasons.

Dr. McClenahan points out that between 1958 and 1963 the population of our country rose about 14.3 per cent, but the amount of x-ray film shipped (a good test of numbers of x-rays being taken) rose some 44 per cent. He urges that the only way diagnostic x-rays can be kept safe is to emphasize the word "necessary" when x-rays are ordered, and to forget the word "routine." Finally, he urges doctors to think of what actual difference an x-ray will make in their care of the particular patient—in which case Dave's internist would have ordered *no* x-rays at all!

Why You Must Be Careful of X-rays

The answer here is one word: cancer. With a competent radiologist there need be no fear of such tragedies as we have seen when a non-radiologist—a G.P. or internist or whatever—starts using a machine for which he's not fully trained. But we are only beginning to learn the damage that can result when radiation— what x-rays really are—is promiscuously or unnecessarily or even "safely" (by current standards) employed. Certainly the most complete and largest investigations so far on the effects of radiation in producing leukemia in human beings are those carried out by the Atomic Bomb Casualty Commission on the victims of our A-bombs dropped at Hiroshima and Nagasaki.

Age here was clearly a factor, with the highest risk of developing leukemia being found in children under the age of ten. One thing that has been proven experimentally beyond question is that cancers of nearly every tissue of the body can be produced by radiation. The World War II atomic bombs have now been shown to produce cancers other than leukemia, although it took these other types of cancer more time to develop.

Recent studies have revealed other disturbing—and, hopefully, preventive—facts. In a careful comparison of healthy children with children dying of leukemia, it was found that those who had been exposed to x-rays while still in the uterus had almost double the frequency of leukemia. In fact, all cancers increased under these conditions, and it's been found that the increased cancer risk was directly proportional to the number of the x-rays taken of the pregnant mother, about a 50 per cent increase in all cancers, according to one report. Lung cancers, breast cancers, even cancers of the thyroid have been reported as resulting from radiation, and it's becoming clearer that even low levels of radiation can produce cancers. The importance of using the specialist, who alone is likely to keep up to the minute on problems in his field, is clear.

Dr. Irwin Bross, chief epidemiologist at New York State's famed cancer center, Roswell Park Memorial Institute, has discovered that the so-called safe levels for radiation are not necessarily safe. Evidently even the low levels used for pregnant women are enough to increase the risk of cancer ten times in some children, and Dr. Bross has urged an immediate revision of our standards and levels of x-ray dosage. The non-radiologist isn't likely to be right up to date on information of this sort, or to have the training needed for applying such new and technical data.

How to Control Your Own Medical Radiation

This is a matter of managing your doctor. The minute he starts talking about or ordering x-rays, it's time for you to ask, "For what purpose do you want the x-rays, Doctor?" And if you hear the word "routine" in his answer, prepare to say "no," quietly but firmly and repeatedly. The so-called routine x-ray is deeply objected to by conscientious and competent radiologists such as Dr. McClenahan.

You can best counter the "routine x-ray" bit from your own doctor with another question: "But are these x-rays *really* necessary?" Had Dave done this with his internist, he might have ended up without unnecessary radiation. X-rays are often taken "for future reference" or "because we don't have the earlier ones." But even when x-rays are missing, their interpretation by a radiologist should be available—and this report will serve just as well, unless there is a really urgent reason for repeating the film.

This is particularly important on entering a hospital, where some staff doctors will automatically order flocks of x-rays. To protect yourself, you have to question virtually every x-ray, and you're likely to find the radiologist on your side. In fact, you can ask this specialist how many of the films ordered actually will be of any value to diagnosis or treatment, and which will merely be different ways of looking at the same thing.

There is one last pair of questions which you must ask, loudly and clearly and often: "If you have this x-ray or set of x-rays, will it add anything to the knowledge you already have? What difference will all these x-rays actually make in what is decided for me?" You'll quickly know whether your exposure to possible radiation damage is warranted by the possible benefits. If you look back at some of the problems we've discussed, you'll see how these questions would have prevented them.

Who Should Take the X-rays and Why?

We've already seen what happens when non-radiologists get involved in taking x-rays. When your doctor wants to take x-rays himself, you can protect yourself with a frank but friendly question: "Have you had special training in radiology, Doctor?" If his answer is "no," so should yours be to the x-rays. If he answers "yes," then ask: "Who will interpret these films?" If the doctor intends to do it himself—particularly if he's had no special training and isn't currently in radiology—you should have serious doubts about what he's proposing and about him as your doctor.

According to radiologists, there is one exception to the rule that non-specialists should never interpret x-rays. The orthopedic surgeon (who specializes in fractured bones and other musculo-skeletal problems) is usually well qualified to read an x-ray of a broken bone, and the fact that he can do so immediately is valuable. But once the orthopedic surgeon gets beyond a routine fracture—say, into obscure bone diseases or complex spinal x-rays—he too is out of his depth and better off leaving interpretation to the radiologists.

The radiologist himself should have his boards, just as any other specialist does, and the tests of his quality roughly follow those of other doctors. The ones in university teaching hospitals are usually best, because so many people are looking over their shoulders in the essentially academic atmosphere. The quality of a radiologist tends—all other things being equal—to follow the quality of his hospital, and for this you can look back to our chapter on hospitals. The quality of the private radiologist is difficult to judge—another evidence of the importance of a good family doctor, for he's in a better position to evaluate, simply by having used this specialist.

A study by the Gynecologic Department of Roswell Park Memorial Institute some years ago is most revealing—and a shocking illustration of the need to be knowledgeable in your choice of health care, for your life's sake. Cancer of the uterine cervix is not easy to treat, and in some parts of Europe only special clinics are permitted to handle this problem.

A Roswell Park medical team studied the effectiveness of the radiation treatment of this cancer by comparing the results achieved by a specialized cancer hospital (Roswell Park), 5 teaching hospitals of medical schools in upper New York State, 21 non-teaching hospitals (located in these same cities), and 106 community hospitals. Since cancer is reportable in New York State, more than nine out of ten cases are listed in the state registry. These hospitals' records for 1949 and 1959 were checked and each individual case reviewed, follow-ups done, and all patients' names checked in the State Death Rolls.

The exact results are too detailed for this book, but in general followed the pattern seen in 1959: the survival rate in the cancer hospital was 57 per cent, compared with 28 per cent in the teaching hospitals, 23 per cent in the non-teaching hospitals, and only 19 per cent in the community hospitals. Yet the cancer hospital treated the worst problems, the teaching hospitals the next to worst, and so on down the line.

Clearly, you want specialized care for difficult disorders, but cancer hospitals are unique among hospitals both in their relative rarity and in the disease they fight. Here it's possible to get the experts (in this case, radiologists) who see far more of these problems than anyone else and so have greater experience and expertise. The result is that only one-third the number of patients survived this cancer in the community hospitals as in the cancer hospitals—which evidently didn't stop the less-qualified doctors or hospitals from continuing to treat such cases. The only protection *you* have is the way *you* manage your health care. Again, though, you see how university teaching hospitals are better than any others except the ultra-specialized cancer hospital (a unique situation).

The Special Problem in Dental X-rays

Dental x-rays are less powerful than medical x-rays and therefore less dangerous, but the danger is still there. When having dental x-rays taken, you should be protected with a lead apron, and you can ask about the speed of the dental x-ray films. This should be the fastest type, underexposed and overdeveloped to further reduce radiation (for more details, see Chapter 7). The so-called full-mouth x-ray series is usually eighteen films, but it shouldn't be done more often than every two years unless very special problems warrant it. The use of hand and eye and a little effort can cut even the so-called bite-wings (four or six x-rays), which show decay alone, so that once a year becomes sufficient instead of the routine six months.

There are new machines that make possible an x-ray with a single exposure or two, but these are still too rare to be worth more than a mention. But the information already discussed indicates clearly that great hesitation must be used before x-raying the teeth of a pregnant woman or of a child—and these should be done *only* if a lead apron is used. Outlaw the word "routine" and demand personal consideration for *your* needs, *your* personal requirements, not just an automatic treatment like everyone else's. Otherwise, the dentist is so accustomed to think in terms of x-rays that he will overuse them without recognizing the hazards involved.

The only protection against the abuse of dental x-rays is *you* —your awareness of the dangers and your insistence on protection and reduced exposure.

Points to Remember

1. Wherever possible, x-rays should be taken only by a radiologist or by a technician under the close supervision of a radiologist. Only the radiologist should "read" the x-ray.

2. When any non-radiologist wants to take an x-ray of you —your G.P. or internist or whoever—ask if he's had special training in radiology and whether he has a radiologist check on his interpretation, to make sure nothing is missed. If his answers aren't "yes," you are being subjected to radiation unnecessarily.

3. The one exception is that an orthopedic surgeon is likely to be entirely competent to interpret an x-ray of a broken bone, and save you time and trouble.

4. For radiation therapy in cancer, it's safest to turn to specialized cancer hospitals, whose experience and expertise markedly improve chances of survival. University teaching hospitals get the next best results, but it's dangerous to consider anything else. In one study cancer hospitals gave double the survival rate of the next best, the university teaching hospitals.

5. Never permit "routine" or "just to be sure" or "for the record" x-rays—there should be a distinct reason. No x-ray should be taken unless it materially contributes to the treatment or handling of your problem, or makes a diagnosis feasible which otherwise would not be possible.

6. Dental full-mouth x-ray series should be done no oftener than every two years unless there is special reason. "Bite-wings" usually need be done only once a year if a careful oral examination is carried out every six months.

7. Special precautions must be taken to protect children and pregnant women from unnecessary x-rays.

9

The Medical Drug Scene, the Doctor, and You

The medical drug scene has turned into a drug game: with "drug" meant in its true sense of "medication for the treatment of disease" (narcotics and heroin or marijuana are only one part), and "game" used in the sense of the late Dr. Eric Berne's book on transactional analysis, *Games People Play.*

This drug game is a complex and all too often life-threatening matter, resulting in pill-popping, drug-taking, and drug-seeking (addictive) behavior. It's produced through the collaboration, conscious or unconscious, of the various people who play it in a series of ever-changing combinations—doctor and patient, pharmacist and pharmaceutical (drug) company, hospital and clinic. The only character in this dangerous charade who is always present—who foots the bill and pays the price, however high, in money or health or life itself—is *you,* the patient, the drug-taker.

Underlying the whole drug game is simply money. Were it not for the economic features of our health-care and industrial systems, there would be no need for this or the following chapters. Managing the drug scene would merely be a matter of seeing to it that your doctor knew his business. But here, as in so many facets of our lives, money enters one phase of the situation and manages to contaminate everything involved in it. In this chapter you'll find the techniques and information you need in order to win this deadly game and to protect both your health and your pocket. Virtually every one of us is involved in the drug game—and not just once or twice but many times in the course of our lives.

The Drug Game and the Price You Pay, Physically and Financially

The drug game is compounded of numerous factors: the over-use or underuse of drugs; the use of drugs that by themselves or in mixtures are of no value or are dangerous; the administration of numbers or combinations of drugs that can cause serious and even life-threatening reactions. The frequency of adverse drug reactions has become a national health problem of the first magnitude. Just look at the figures: 1.5 million hospital admissions *every year* are estimated to be caused by adverse drug reactions, and the hospital stay of these patients is some 40 per cent longer than the average.

Dr. Donald C. Brodie, professor of pharmacy at the University of California Medical School, San Francisco, puts the cost of hospitalization because of drug reactions at almost $1 billion (not counting the expenses of diagnosis and treatment). He further reports a study by Dr. James A. Visconti at the University of Mississippi Teaching Hospital in which the direct and indirect costs incurred by 41 patients admitted for drug reactions ran to $116,835. And how do you figure the cost to lives? From 1949 to 1965 the reported number of annual deaths from adverse drug reactions rose from under 200 to over 500. Clearly, these figures are on the rise, with no end in sight.

Studies reporting these tragic figures come from coast to coast and border to border, from Canada and from across the seas. The drug problem seems to be assuming epidemic proportions, and it is likely that, iceberg-style, there may be a great deal more under the surface. Many drug-reaction problems aren't reported for one of two reasons: either the victim has taken some over-the-counter (OTC) medication, feels guilty because the reaction is his own fault, and so conceals it; or the physician may not want to admit that his prescription (Rx) caused illness because it will show his ignorance of the correct drug therapy (treatment) or might hurt his reputation or expose him to the malpractice suit he fears so much.

Leaders of the medical profession—public health doctors, epidemiologists, teachers of medicine, internists, pediatricians, and others—are becoming increasingly concerned over the drug-reaction problem. Studies have revealed adverse reactions in from 10 to 30 per cent of hospital patients (and no one knows how many in private offices). Some 5 per cent of *all* admissions to the medical sections of general hospitals are due to serious drug reactions, and a recent federal report puts the annual cost of these adverse reactions at some $3 billion.

But how about you and me? A very revealing recent study of 75 representative patients selected by scientific methods was done at the University of Florida Teaching Hospital in Gainesville. The medical team—Dr. Leighton E. Cluff and Dr. Ronald B. Stewart—found that more than half these people reported adverse reactions to one or more drugs at some time. Moreover, 16 per cent had had reactions to more than one drug, and 4 patients had had reactions to as many as four drugs. These reactions varied: Ann passed out after taking codeine for a sprained back; Joan had a severe stomach hemorrhage from a few aspirins; some unfortunate patients developed severe blood diseases and other fatal reactions.

The most serious adverse drug reactions arise from the self-admitted weaknesses and errors of the medical profession. To protect yourself you must learn to manage your doctor in the medication area as well as the other areas discussed in this book. However, self-medication is an established American pattern—and probably a necessity under our health-care system—so it might be wise to look at this aspect of the problem first.

You and the Medicines You Need

A recent Louis Harris poll revealed that two-thirds of Americans believe they are well informed about health care, while only slightly more than a quarter feel they don't get enough information. But when pollsters asked the public specific questions about sickness and health, an information gap quickly appeared. While nearly two-thirds of the public said they could recognize the symptoms of the most serious diseases, nearly one-third didn't know a single one of the seven danger signals of cancer and only one-sixth could identify even one. As for heart attacks and heart conditions, the great fear and number-one killer of our time, more than one-quarter couldn't identify a single symptom, while only half could offer more than one.

It is by knowing such information that you can gain an understanding of how to manage your doctor; with this awareness you can shore up your defenses against ill health, while assuring yourself of good medical care when the need arises. In more than one way, the most important fact revealed by this Harris poll is how the public gets its health information: primarily, from its doctors. This would be fine except for the low level of knowledge of drug therapy among doctors, and the fact that the survey showed inadequate contact between people and doctors. Fewer than three out of four people see a doctor even five times a year, and about one in eight never visits a doctor's office.

Next to the doctor, the most common source of health information is television commercials, followed by the medical columns in newspapers or medical sections in magazines, medical news on TV, and newspaper and magazine advertising. But before you condemn the gullible public, remember that the physician too depends on advertising for drug information. In fact, most doctors look to the drug-company advertisements in medical magazines (many of which are non-scientific and distributed free, thanks to their large volume of these very ads). "Detail men," the sales representatives of the drug manufacturers, spend their days visiting doctors' offices to promote their products and leave samples, in the hope that the doctor will use their particular brand. These men are usually neither pharmacists nor physicians, yet they commonly get calls late at night or during weekends from distraught doctors seeking their advice on how to treat a particular medical problem. The strength of these commercial influences can't be fully appreciated unless you visit the drug-company booths at medical conventions and see their giveaways and the crowds of doctors around them (much larger than those at the scientific exhibits).

Over-the-Counter (OTC) Drugs

You—the patient, the consumer, the drug-taker—are faced with a two-sided drug problem. First comes the matter of self-medication, which is essential to our entire health-care system. For this you must examine the OTC drugs available in neighborhood drugstores and supermarkets. You also must learn to manage your doctor, for the more dangerous drugs are the ones he prescribes for more serious conditions (heart disease and infections, for example).

If you are confused by the OTC products on pharmacy shelves, you are not alone. Dr. Charles C. Edwards, until recently commissioner of the Food and Drug Administration (FDA), points out that there are an estimated 100,000 to 500,000 separate OTC drugs. The National Academy of Sciences/National Research Council (NAS/NRC), in its Drug Efficacy Study, found that a mere 400 products could be chosen to be broadly representative of this whole range of products—and that there were actually only some 200 significant active ingredients in these hundreds of thousands of OTC drugs!

Dr. Edwards reported to Senator Gaylord Nelson's Subcommittee on Monopoly that this NAS/NRC study found 85 per cent of our OTC drugs could *not* be proven effective, judging from the 400 representative ones. A bare 27 per cent were *probably* effective (additional evidence will be needed to prove their effectiveness); 47 per cent were *possibly* effective (no evidence of effectiveness was available); and 11 per cent were ineffective. This left only 15 per cent that actually proved useful.

Information on the effectiveness of the OTC drugs will be published as the NAS/NRC studies are completed. Clearly, self-medication requires a good deal of information on your part, and also runs head on into deeply ingrained health attitudes, beliefs, and practices.

You and Super-Health

Before World War II, even taking an aspirin was a big thing and called for consultation. But with the advent of our many powerful and effective drugs, from antibiotics to tranquilizers, from polio vaccines to L-dopa and the steroids, the average household is now accustomed to seeing medication, pills, and capsules being taken by every member of the family—for both valid and invalid reasons.

A very recent report made with the cooperation of seven federal agencies (coordinated by the FDA) revealed some startling insights into Americans' use of drugs—most important, the strange quest of the public for some sort of "super-health." Where doctors see good health as the absence of illness, many Americans regard it as some sort of Nirvana in which the person has unlimited strengths and energies, no tension or anxiety or depression, only an almost other-worldly happiness and peace. Since this feeling won't happen naturally, people think that it can be brought about through the magic of special foods and nutrition.

Millions of Americans clearly base their health decisions on the belief that "anything is worth a try." Many believe that there are so many individual differences among us that almost any treatment, no matter how irrational or far out, may be beneficial to someone. This trial-and-error approach to medical problems must be the major reason behind the plethora of questionable health practices. The FDA survey found that 50 million adults wouldn't be convinced even by virtually unanimous expert opinions that any hypothetical "cancer cure" was worthless. Three-quarters of the American public believe that extra vitamins provide more pep and energy; one-fifth believes that even diseases such as arthritis and cancer are the result, at least in part, of taking nutritional supplements without a doctor's advice.

In 1971 the public spent more than $210 million for OTC laxatives and other elimination aids. The FDA study found that two-thirds of the adults believe a bowel movement every day is necesssary for health (it isn't), while nearly one-third believe it's appropriate to do something regularly to help with bowel movements. Some 2.5 million adults take something every day to help with bowel movements.

Some 16 million adults medicate themselves without seeing a doctor, including 11 million arthritis sufferers, who turn to a variety of aids, from joint lubricators to diets and copper bracelets. Potentially the most dangerous self-medication of all is practiced by the 16 million adults who report having arthritis, rheumatism, asthma, allergies, hemorrhoids, heart trouble, high blood pressure, or diabetes, and who have never been diagnosed by a doctor. As the Senate Subcommittee on Consumer Interests of the Elderly concluded after studying the FDA findings: "It became apparent during the hearings that quackery persists in the nation because of puzzling consumer attitudes, even when facts are readily available."

One thing is clear. You must be able to turn to your doctor for accurate, authoritative advice. But first you must learn to manage your doctor.

You and Your Doctor: OTC *vs.* Rx

There are major differences between the OTC drugs and the ones your doctor prescribes for you. Perhaps most important, the OTC drugs are generally for the relief of symptoms (headache, heartburn, menstrual pain, sunburn, etc.), while your doctor's prescription (Rx) is aimed at diseases (high blood pressure, infections, glaucoma, etc.).

OTC drugs are a little like old shoes—safe, comfortable, familiar. They involve minimal risk and usually contain long-used components that are well understood and have a fairly high degree of safety. You can usually tell when OTC drugs give you help: the headache is relieved, the heartburn easier, the sunburn less painful, the cough better.

Prescription drugs, on the other hand, are tricky to assess, and with serious conditions it's dangerous for the patient to try. Moreover, these drugs are more potent and by their very nature more toxic ("poisonous"); when the competent doctor prescribes them, he weighs the possible benefit against the risk involved. It's like a balance sheet—side effects, toxicity, and risk on one side, benefit to be gained on the other. Sometimes potentially deadly drugs are tried when life hangs in the balance, when the gamble is for a life otherwise lost.

How much of the drugs used by the American public are OTC and how much Rx? In terms of dollars, the Social Security Administration found that during 1969 Americans spent $2.6 billion for OTC drugs and $4 billion for prescriptions—both figures virtually double what they had been ten years earlier. While no one can tell how many OTC items are sold annually, we do know (from data in medical, hospital, and druggist magazines) that in 1969 some 1,866 million prescriptions were filled in the United States (30 per cent of these were filled for hospitalized patients).

With this kind of money at stake, it's obvious why pharmaceutical houses are constantly jockeying for position—sending out detail men to visit physicians, giving out gimmicks, hosting physicians at conventions, footing the bill for coffee and entertainment at medical society meetings. Dr. Richard P. Penna, of the American Pharmaceutical Association, estimates that Americans spent some $557 million for OTC analgesics (painkillers) in 1969, while the industry put some $102 million into advertising these drugs.

Observers have noted repeatedly that after ten years or so of general practice, doctors utilize less and less of what they learned in medical school—which is ten years out of date anyway. Many busy and harried doctors cannot find the time to read medical journals, and increasingly their source of information becomes the drug detail men.

Overprescribing and Addiction

The real problem in the drug game is the unfortunate combination of the doctor's weaknesses and desires, the patient's problems and pill-popping way of life, and the high-pressure promotion behind modern drugs. Dr. Donald Brodie, professor of pharmacy at the University of California, San Francisco, clearly expresses our urgent need of controls over drug utilization because of ". . . a general misuse of many drugs, the apparent irresponsible prescribing habits of many physicians . . . and a certain psychological dependence that society in general has on drugs."

The facts are there in Dr. Brodie's quotations from a paper given by Dr. Harry F. Dowling, who revealed how investigators in one study found virtually 40 per cent of doctors pushed into using a new drug by the pressure exerted by the seller. In another survey more than two-thirds of the doctors were influenced this way, and most of them considered the promotional materials of the drug houses twice as important as the drug information coming to them from their professional colleagues.

The widespread problem of overprescribing is well known. Many observers of the medical scene recognize it as one of the primary.causes of drug addiction (we shall go into this in Chapter 12). The introduction of new drugs dropped sharply with the passage of the Kefauver-Harris Acts of 1962, from 250 in 1962 to 80 only four years later and 62 in 1969, but 1970 saw a rise to 105. There are still lots of new drugs that, under our system, the drug companies have to push to make money.

Before you ask your doctor for an Rx, remember that drugs really aren't magic. Many new drugs come and go, but few ever become permanent useful additions to a doctor's armamentarium. With all the wonder drugs introduced for headaches, there are virtually only two (and one is aspirin) that have stood the test of time for efficacy and safety. Over the last two decades there has been a steady parade of drugs to relieve rheumatoid arthritis, from the cortico-steroids (such as cortisone) to phenylbutazone, hydrochloroquine, indomethacin, DMSO—but aspirin still remains the cornerstone of drug therapy.

Recognizing the Doctor Who Overprescribes

In hearings before the Senate Subcommittee on Monopoly, Dr. Paul D. Stolley, professor of epidemiology at Johns Hopkins School of Hygiene and Public Health, pointed out that nearly two-thirds of all common colds treated with medication by doctors were really being mistreated. And the committee received testimony about the case of a patient who actually died from the inappropriate use of an antibiotic for the common cold! This wasn't malicious—the doctor just didn't know. But *your* job is to protect yourself with the right information.

The physician that Dr. Stolley termed "the less appropriate prescriber" presented a surprising picture in this study, whose results may serve as a warning for you. "This less appropriate prescriber did not have a larger, more hurried practice . . . but tended to have a smaller practice. . . . He generally trusted the information he received from the detail man and looked forward to his visits; as a solo practitioner in a small town, it may have been one of the few sources of professional contact that he experienced. . . . [He] tended to refer his patients to other physicians less and had fewer patients referred to him than his colleagues. . . . He also attended fewer medical meetings. . . ."

It's interesting to note that the questions and tests suggested in our chapter on finding a family doctor are likely to eliminate just such a practitioner and protect you. But there is also an economic factor that drives the doctor and the attitudes of the public to make this overuse of drugs possible.

How You Can Avoid Overprescribing

The doctor has a limited time for each patient if he wants to provide that fur coat for his wife, school for his children, and an extra car. If he allows too much time for each patient he'll have to raise his fees, so instead he tries to fit as many patients as possible into a given time slot. He cuts visits short in a way that is satisfying both to him and to his patients: he writes out a prescription.

Both doctor and patient are already oriented to "doing something" for complaints. The patient will feel cheated if he is told, "Go home, take an aspirin, and rest"; he will feel he's not getting anything for his money. But if he walks out carrying a prescription, he feels he's been given something, something's been done, he's got his money's worth. He may even express it when he comes in: "Doc, do something for this cold—an injection or prescription or something."

Walk in that way and the doctor who can't spare the time to educate you in why he should do nothing, afraid you'll compare him to the doctor down the block who pours out the Rx for green or yellow or whatever capsules, gives you an Rx to keep you as a patient and ends the visit in as short a time as possible. And besides, the detail man may just have left some new samples ... So you leave with your Rx, and you've played your part in the drug game.

The Problem of Drug Interactions

The quantity of drugs prescribed or taken without doctors' orders is overwhelming, and the number of interactions between these powerful chemicals is increasing at a rate that has experts deeply concerned. With 1.5 million hospital admissions, the number of resulting deaths may soon approach 1,000 or more a year unless we take protective action.

The fact that physicians fail to educate the public, which naturally turns to them for health information, is a result of the economics of the doctor's time and the cause of one of the problems of drug interactions. In the study made by Dr. Ronald B. Stewart and Dr. Leighton E. Cluff, their 75 subjects took a total of 245 Rx drugs, only one-third of which could be correctly identified by the patients. Only a little over two-thirds of the patients felt they received adequate information from their doctors as to what the drug was for and how to use it.

To make matters worse, virtually all the patients taking prescribed drugs were also taking OTC ones. One patient had taken

14 drugs in the thirty-day period studied, another took 13, two others each used 11. Patients received an average of 9.5 separate chemicals during the thirty-day period studied—one had taken 28, while eight had taken 20 or more. With more than half the patients reporting previous adverse drug reactions, a study revealed the possibility of drug interactions in more than half the cases—a sad commentary on the care and expertise exercised by the prescribing doctors. Hospital charts rarely show fewer than 10 to 15 drugs during a patient's stay, and one professor of medicine reported that one patient's chart listed 43 drugs!

A recent computer study of prescriptions given some 42,000 Californians showed 84 per cent of the patients being given Rx that presented serious problems of drug interactions. More than half those getting blood thinners (for heart conditions or strokes) were given Rx for other drugs capable of serious interactions; one-third of those on anti-diabetic drugs were given other medication that either antagonized or exaggerated the diabetes-control drug; more than one-quarter of those getting drugs to control blood chemistry got antagonizing medicines; and three-quarters of those getting digitalis and water pills (for heart or kidney conditions) were not given the supplements needed and without which fatal effects can occur.

Managing Your
Doctor, Hospital, Pharmacist, and Drugs

Managing your doctor really consists of absorbing all these stories and facts, so that you will know how to react effectively when you next see your doctor. First you must honestly ask yourself why you're visiting that doctor—do you really want help for a life-problem (your marriage or job or whatever)? And how do you handle your OTC medication? Are you seeking "super-health"? Do you turn to drug ads for advice on health care? Or are you prepared to seek the best modern medicine has to offer, even if it's just the advice to go home and rest and maybe take an aspirin?

If you're sincerely interested in what's best for you, you'll visit a doctor if you want to, but then you will avoid pushing him. Doctors push easily, and if he suspects you want something, he'll give it to you—and you'll pay for it both in money and, much more important, in health. Don't ever say: "Doc, my friend had a cold like this and his doctor gave him a shot and it cleared up—I want one." If you do, you're just asking for trouble. The right approach is: "I've got this cold, I feel miserable—what do *you* advise?" Or, perhaps, to play it doubly safe: "Doctor, I've got a terribly uncomfortable cold—what do you advise? Should I just go home and sweat it out?"

If, despite all these precautions, your doctor suddenly pulls out his pen and an Rx pad, you had better take over promptly to protect yourself, because that Rx may be a simple reflex action, the only way he knows to end a visit or a discussion. Ask quickly: "What is that medication, Doctor?" And if the answer doesn't tell you everything about both the drug and why you need it, then go on with: "Is it really necessary? Exactly what do you expect it to accomplish, and are there any side effects? Can I expect any reactions?"

The next step depends on your doctor's response. If it's not satisfactory, you must probe on: "Tell me, Doctor, is there any alternative medication? Is there any professional disagreement about the wisdom of using this drug for my problem?" If you are to take the drug for any length of time you must also ask: "What precautions must I take? Should I check back with you for any special tests?" (Some medication should be followed with regular blood tests.) "When should I stop taking it?"

Finally, any other medication (aspirin, laxatives, antacids, *anything* you take regularly or even occasionally) should be checked with him to prevent an interaction. Also, ask about any other Rx medicine he's given you—he may not remember what he gave you before, but if he can't tell immediately by looking at your chart there's something very wrong. The doctor should have every medication he's prescribed on your record. In fact, it might not be a bad idea to double-check a new Rx with your pharmacist, because if he's competent in his field he's probably more familiar with drugs and their incompatibilities than your doctor.

Increasingly, both hospitals and doctors are urging more dependency on pharmacists to protect patients from prescription errors. For this reason it's good to use the same pharmacist regularly so he has a record of all your Rx. Enlisting your pharmacist's help in your health care may well prove rewarding in protecting yourself.

Even in the hospital you have to take responsibility for your own health protection. Your drug safety depends on the quality of the hospital (in Chapter 3 we've discussed in detail the ways of judging these). The larger academic hospitals are increasingly using pharmacologists and pharmacists to control the problem because the traditional hospital methods of drug distribution and use are distressingly error-prone. Dr. Brodie calls attention to a study of the existing system at the University of Arkansas Medical Center (since it's in an academic setting it should be one of our better hospitals): investigators found an error rate of from 11 to 19 per cent.

In the hospital, too, you will have to depend on yourself. When the nurse arrives with your medication and calls your name, identify yourself with a loud "yes." If she wants to see your name bracelet, stick out your arm to make it easier for her to check it against your medicine card. But if you think she's not following your doctor's orders, don't hesitate to ask, politely but definitely. Learn to recognize the medicine your doctor has ordered and talk to him about it: "What is that white pill with the pink band?"—or the green capsule or the blue liquid. Find out what he's giving you, how often, and why; that way you can check what you're getting. Your doctor's not likely to change your medication without mentioning it to you; when he does, ask what the new stuff will be like—color, shape, and form (capsule, tablet, or liquid)—to make sure you don't continue getting the old drug or a new but incorrect one.

Finally, tell the nurse if you feel funny or get any strange reactions from medication. Harry took months getting over the itching and peeling of his hands and feet because he thought the penicillin he was taking would help his brain abscess. He felt he should accept the discomfort for the sake of the greater advantage of controlling his infection. Only when a neurologist noticed the raw patches on arms and legs due to the scratching (busy doctors in a big hospital look only to their specialized concerns) was a new antibiotic used. Harry's complaint would have sacrificed nothing in infection-fighting but would have saved him months of misery.

Always remember, nurses and other hospital personnel don't ask questions to be pleasant. Mark always had a cheery "I'm fine, thank you" when his nurse asked how he was feeling. Then one day he had to be rushed to emergency surgery for a perforated stomach ulcer—he never mentioned the severe pain he was having despite the medication and care. When medical people ask you questions, they do so to help and protect you; cooperate by telling the exact truth, not by "being nice."

In larger and university teaching hospitals, pharmacists and clinical pharmacologists are being increasingly used to control drug-reaction problems. Even in community hospitals new and original ideas are being tried by forward-looking professionals. Dr. Brodie tells of an experiment that may prove a model for the country. In the Charlottesville, Virginia, area, physicians and pharmacists have joined together so that the practicing pharmacists routinely check all prescriptions and call the doctor if there is any question about the drug prescribed, its dosage, or the form in which it's been ordered. They also review with the patient the doctor's instruction about the medicine, its use, and so on.

To protect yourself under this haphazard system of ours, you, the patient, must effect your own drug control. You must take the responsibility of managing your doctor, hospital, and pharmacist, in addition to guarding yourself against misuse of OTC drugs.

Points to Remember

1. If you experience an adverse drug reaction, report it to your family doctor and your regular pharmacist. They can serve and protect you better if they have this information.

2. Neither drugs nor nutritional supplements can give you "super-health." Since 85 per cent of OTC drugs have *no* adequate proof of their effectiveness, it's best to be conservative in their use rather than expose yourself to the possibility of adverse drug reactions. The FDA constantly brings out new reports on the effectiveness of OTC drugs. These are worth keeping up with and noting for future reference.

3. OTC drugs really aren't there to "cure" anything; they're meant for the relief of symptoms. For cures you have to turn to the doctor, with far more potent, and dangerous, prescription drugs, to be used after his skilled diagnosis and under his direction.

4. Physicians tend to be inadequate at understanding and handling drugs. *You* must be on the alert to prevent problems, and the best way is to find a good family doctor.

5. Part of the problem of overprescribing is *you*. Visit your doctor and let him know you want him to "do something" for every complaint, and he will: he'll give you an Rx for which you're likely to pay both in money and in health.

6. When you see your doctor, *ask:* "What is best done for this problem?" When an Rx is offered: "What is the medication? Is it really necessary? . . . What will it do? Are there any side effects? . . . Is there any alternative medicine? How much professional agreement is there on its use?" Don't forget: "What precautions should I take? When should I check back with you? . . . How long do I take it?"

7. Always tell your doctor *any* other drugs you're taking, no matter what.

8. If your doctor offers an Rx, check on him by asking about previous drugs he's prescribed for you. He should have the time, drug, and all other details precisely recorded on your chart, or it's time to seek another doctor. Find out whether you can or should continue taking it.

9. When you're in the hospital, learn from your doctor what the shape, form, and color of your medication is and the times you're supposed to get it. If something doesn't seem right, *ask!* If you have any strange reaction to the drug, tell the nurse and the doctor.

10. Your pharmacist can be a great help. He should know which drugs are incompatible and give adverse reactions. In general, the pharmacist should know more about drugs and their reactions than the doctors.

And now for the specifics—first, the "miracle" drugs.

10

Guarding against the Miracle Drugs that Spell "Murder"

A healthy twenty-five-year-old man had a sore throat. His doctor prescribed an antibiotic called chloramphenicol (trade name: Chloromycetin) for nine days. Within two months the young man developed aplastic anemia (a blood disorder that kills the majority of its victims), and within four months, he was dead.

A forty-nine-year-old man with a middle-ear infection was given this same antibiotic for only five days. He too developed aplastic anemia within four months.

Neither of these conditions should have been treated with chloramphenicol. The dangers of this drug were well known to knowledgeable physicians, widely reported, and information on it was available in AMA publications and elsewhere.

In *The Medicine Man*, the late Dr. Leonard Tushnet told of a young man with a sore throat who was given a shot of penicillin by his doctor. The throat improved, but the drug produced hives. So he was given an antihistamine, but that made him sleepy, and he cut his hand at work. The medical department applied an ointment that contained penicillin, and the serious reaction to it was treated with steroid drugs, which caused a stomach ulcer and hemorrhaging. Part of the young man's stomach was removed, but an infection was treated with antibiotics that caused diarrhea. Medication for this interfered with his vision; the young man's car smashed into a tree, and he was killed. Dr. Tushnet vouched for the truth of this story!

None of these tales is in the least surprising to those familiar with the antibiotic scene in medical care. Penicillin alone causes reactions in 9 or 10 per cent of patients and takes 100 to 300 lives annually in the United States. Figures in this field are notoriously hard to come by because the evidence of antibiotic reactions isn't always clear and doctors are afraid to identify their Rx as the cause of a reaction for fear of a malpractice suit.

As Dr. Stolley has pointed out, most sore throats are actually virus infections, which cannot be treated or "cured" by any antibiotics or antibacterial drugs (such as the sulfas).

What does all this mean to you? Let's look at the statistics and then see how you can use this information to help you protect yourself against the widespread dangers we have seen.

What Are the Figures?

The Food and Drug Administration is deeply concerned, because one in every five prescriptions given to Americans is for an antibiotic. This would be fine—if there were a valid or safe reason for even half these prescriptions (almost 400 million Rx were filled in 1970). But a recent study by Dr. James A. Visconti, director of Ohio State University Hospitals Drug Information Center, and Andrew W. Roberts is shocking: in a 500-bed community hospital, Dr. Visconti found that one-third of the more than 1,000 patients admitted during a one-month period were given antibacterial drugs. Taking an HEW Task Force definition of rational prescribing as "the appropriate selection of . . . the right drug for the right patient in the right amounts at the right time," Dr. Visconti found that less than 13 per cent of the antibiotics in the community hospital investigated were actually prescribed rationally. Of those getting these drugs, some 15 per cent suffered adverse reactions. The tragedy: some 92 per cent of the adverse reactions were among those patients whose Rx were found to be irrational or questionable. Financially, too, the study discovered disaster, for barely 9 per cent (less than $1,700) of the more than $18,000 spent on the drugs was for rational prescriptions.

Other studies, both in university teaching hospitals and in a group of community hospitals, have found that from one-half to two-thirds of the prescriptions for antimicrobial drugs were irrational; either the patient needed no such treatment or the dosage was inappropriate or inadequate.

How Miraculous Are the "Miracle" Drugs?

Dr. Leighton Cluff, professor of medicine at Gainesville's University of Florida College of Medicine, bluntly told Senator Nelson's Subcommittee on Monopoly: "The public is generally unaware of the limited effectiveness of antibiotics, and often insists or expects physicians to treat any and all presumed infectious diseases with one of these drugs. In part, physicians may be responsible for development of these attitudes...."

It's clear that the antimicrobial drugs cannot help viral infections. Yet Dr. Cluff has found that viral infections are responsible for over 20 per cent of all the illnesses cared for in doctor's offices; among hospitalized patients the proportion is about the same. Acute respiratory infections (the common cold, sore throat, "chest cold," and so on) make up more than one-third of the infections doctors see in their offices, and most are due to viruses. It's long been known that antibiotics are effective only against certain bacteria (each drug has specific bacteria against which it's most effective), and that only laboratory tests can identify the microbe causing the infection and its sensitivity to antibiotic or sulfa drugs. Nevertheless, the detail men urge their use, the physicians in general listen, and the public pays the price in money, in health, and in lives.

What the Doctor Does with Antibiotics

Dr. Stolley and Dr. Louis Lasagna (one of America's great pharmacologists) recently found that 95 per cent of doctors have given one or more prescriptions to patients who had an ordinary cold. Sixty per cent of these were for antibiotics, with penicillin among the most popular. The sulfa drugs also were heavily represented. A recent survey of thirty-seven physicians found they prescribed almost fifty different drugs for the common cold, including nine antibiotics (one of them the deadly chloramphenicol). Dr. Stolley also investigated the antibiotics most frequently prescribed in one county of a mid-Atlantic state; he found that three of the top six were either being attacked by the FDA in an effort to remove them from the market, or had low ratings from the NAS/NRC Drug Efficacy Study (with which doctors should be familiar.

So it's not surprising to find that twenty to fifty tons of penicillin are sold annually in the United States. It's been estimated that one out of every four Americans gets penicillin each year, and that 90 per cent of this is wasted! Dr. Harry F. Dowling, University of Illinois professor emeritus of medicine, told Senator Nelson's Subcommittee that for the fiscal year 1972 the FDA certified enough of the eight most commonly prescribed antibiotics to give fifty doses to every man, woman and child in our country—enough for two sicknesses of average duration. But, as Dr. Dowling emphasized: "It is doubtful that the average person has an illness that requires treatment with an antibiotic more often than once every five or ten years."

This last remark is important for *you*—for how often has your doctor given you an antibiotic?

What You Have to Know about How the Doctor Uses His Miracle Drugs

Here we run into many of the factors mentioned in the last chapter. The Rx is a satisfactory way to end a visit and get on to the next patient, leaving both doctor and patient satisfied that something has been done. The doctor is strongly influenced by your reactions. When you come in expecting medication for the common cold, the physician usually isn't strong enough psychologically or willing to spend the necessary time to tell you the truth. Or perhaps he's just listening to the wrong detail man. As Dr. Dowling has pointed out, detail men succeed in persuading doctors to use new drugs two-thirds or more of the time. Finally, there are the doctor's own fears and anxieties; not certain what's wrong, he plays it safe and prescribes an antibiotic just in case. But he shouldn't use these treacherous drugs "just in case"—only when there's a specific infection and positive diagnosis. If he can't make the diagnosis, he should refer you to someone who can.

The Questions to Ask

To protect yourself, you must always question what is in the Rx your doctor is scribbling out for you. "What are you giving me an antibiotic for, Doc?" And even: "But don't you have to check the germ to make sure that this drug will be effective?" (Yes, there should be a laboratory check so that the correct antibacterial drug is used.) And then you might ask: "I've heard there are some pretty bad side effects from some antibiotics. What can I expect from this one?" (We'll go into adverse reactions shortly.) And then comes the big question: "What would happen, Doctor, if you used conservative treatment and didn't prescribe antibiotic or antibacterial drugs?" This really puts the physician to the test, for conservative therapy will make a common cold disappear as fast as any antimicrobials possibly can!

If you find your doctor admitting that yours is an uncomplicated common cold and he still is giving you an Rx for an antibiotic, look for another physician. If he wants to prescribe chloramphenicol he should have special qualifications in the medical field called "infectious diseases," or else be prepared to show he's capable of handling this deadly drug. Some experts go so far as to feel it should be used only with patients so sick as to require hospitalization.

Now for the details you need to know if you are to manage your doctor—the information you'll need in order to discuss your medical problems with your doctor and find your way through today's health-care maze.

The Adverse Drug Reactions to Miracle Drugs

The famed United States Center for Disease Control (in Atlanta) did a study of prescribing practices in seven community hospitals and found antibiotics being given to about one-third of patients, even though nearly two-thirds of them had *no* documented infections (the urologists were particularly bad in this respect). Dr. Philip R. Lee, professor of social medicine at Los Angeles' University of California School of Medicine, recently recalled a study of fifty-four patients at the University of Southern

California Medical Center: treatment with one of the newest and most expensive antibiotics (cephalexin), which cost an average of $12 a prescription, was revealed to be an irrational therapy for almost all (93 per cent) of the patients for whom it was prescribed. You could have been one of these people—unless you asked why the drug was being given, what were the alternatives, had the diagnosis of "infection" been proven ("documented") by laboratory procedures or a consultation with a specialist in infectious diseases.

It's important to be aware of the variety of reactions people have with these drugs so that as soon as one appears you can inform your doctor. Take Ed, who sat up in bed one morning and got so dizzy that the only way he could get up to call his doctor was to lie down on his stomach and edge off the bed (he couldn't sit up). His antibiotic was immediately discontinued, but since the bacteria causing his infection had been determined, effective substitute antibiotics could be chosen and used without a reaction.

We have already seen that fatal blood disorders can result from misused miracle drugs. Dr. Visconti found that slightly more than half the reactions were gastro-intestinal (nausea and vomiting, diarrhea and distress); slightly more than one-third were allergic (rash, hives, itching); and one-sixth were kidney damage (bloody urine or blood changes). Actually, there is an almost endless number of complications and reactions possible, including damage to the liver or nervous system, kidney failure, blood disorders, disfigurement, disability, and even death. In a recent 500-patient study at Gainesville's University of Florida Medical Center, adverse reactions were found in nearly 40 per cent of the patients, with penicillin and sulfa the worst offenders.

The Super-Infections

When antibacterial drugs are used they eliminate certain microbes, but at the same time they upset nature's balance. On your skin and in your body, in the air you breathe, the food you eat, and the water you drink, there are bacteria that strike up a working relationship with your body—a sort of "live and let live" deal. Such bacteria normally have no ability to "infect" you, to cause that disease process we know as "infection."

Once this natural balance is disturbed, some of the organisms overgrow and a whole host of infections may plague you. These may be as mild as the itching that sometimes appears around the anus after antibiotic therapy, or so severe as to cost the victim his life. The promiscuous use of antibiotics has resulted in an increase of Gram-negative bacteria infections (bacteria are divided into Gram-negative and Gram-positive by the way they react in laboratory tests to the Gram stain). This is a frightening development, for Gram-negative bacteremia (blood poisoning) has a fatality rate, despite antibiotics, of 30 to 50 per cent.

Estimates are that 100,000 to 300,000 Gram-negative bacteremias occur each year. Boston City Hospital showed a 400 per cent increase from 1935 to 1965 (sharply rising from the years before we had antibiotics to today, when we have the miracle drugs).

On top of this problem, some 2 to 7 per cent of hospital patients getting antibiotics also develop some sort of super-infection—perhaps several million people. To this you must add the 500 or 600 million office visits annually, with 60 per cent of those who have respiratory infections getting unnecessary antibiotics—and so you have millions more super-infections.

The Tough New Breed of Bacteria

When you go through a course of antibiotic therapy (a series of penicillin shots or a week or two of sulfa drugs), bacteria on and in your body either are killed off or develop "resistance" to the drug. Should these resistant germs ever win out over the body's natural defenses against infection, that drug to which they're resistant will be of no help in fighting the germs. There is now evidence of such resistance among the germs of gonorrhea, the dreaded "staph," and typhoid. In fact, both of the chief antibiotics used for typhoid are no longer effective against many cases.

Dr. Dowling summed up this typhoid problem: "Where is our security now? Before too long we may be back to the 1930s, when we had no effective therapy for this disease and could only stand by and watch 10 to 15 per cent of the patients die, while others suffered through weeks of serious illness." To protect yourself, you must resist unnecessary antibiotic prescriptions.

The Mystique of the Preventive Antibiotic

One of the major reasons doctors give for using antibiotics is that it will prevent secondary infections such as a sinus or middle-ear infection after a viral disease. This is simply not so. Dr. Stolley knows of *no* scientific evidence for this, and an article in the October 15, 1973, issue of the *Journal of the American Medical Association* by Dr. Benjamin Kagan and Dr. Shirley Fannin, of Los Angeles' University of California School of Medicine, indicates that this "prophylactic" use may lead to more infection than it actually prevents.

The prophylactic use of antibiotics in 130 measles patients resulted in 30 per cent developing secondary bacterial infections; in 298 patients who were not given antibiotics, only 15 per cent developed secondary infections. Among bulbar polio patients, those without miracle drugs developed one-quarter the number of secondary infections of those *with* antibiotics. And bacterial complications were five times as common in surgical patients treated prophylactically as those not given the antibiotics.

True, there are some special cases—people with rheumatic heart disease, for example—where prophylactic use of antibiotics is believed essential. Careful questioning of your doctor should give you the answer, along with some further trust or distrust in the man. The best professional is the one who's not afraid of answering your questions with: "I don't know, but I'll find out and tell you."

The Miracle-Drug Specialists

Specialists in infectious disease are experts in the use of antibiotics, but theirs is a small and relatively new field. It has only a limited number of practitioners, and you are most likely to find them in the university teaching hospitals. These are the doctors who best know how, when, and in what way to use the powerful antimicrobials—unlike the many doctors who are too fast on the draw when it comes to writing an Rx for antibiotics.

Points to Remember

1. Our miracle drugs can kill! Their unnecessary use only makes for trouble.

2. Two-thirds or more oxy prescriptions written for antibiotics are irrational and can only do harm.

3. The common cold and most acute respiratory infections are viral in nature—antibiotics cannot help these.

4. Before an antimicrobial drug is prescribed, the doctor should carry out laboratory procedures to find the infecting germ and which drug it is sensitive to, so that the most effective antibiotic can be used.

5. With 95 per cent of doctors giving a range of fifty different drugs for the common cold, it's best to question such medication carefully.

6. One leading medical expert estimates that the average person has an illness that requires treatment with antibiotics no oftener than once every five or ten years. How often has your doctor given *you* these drugs? Deviation from careful conservative use should have good reason.

7. When you visit your doctor, make it clear you want what's best for you and avoid implying that you want him to do something. If a doctor senses that you want a prescription, he is more likely to give you an antibiotic than any other drug—whether you really need it or not.

8. If an antibiotic is prescribed, *ask* what it is, why it's being given to you, whether the doctor checked to be sure there's an infection, which germ is involved, and whether it's sensitive to antibiotics. You also want to know the possible side effects and what would happen if the doctor used conservative therapy instead of antibacterials.

9. If you get any adverse reactions (some are listed in our chapter, but they are far too numerous and too individual to give them all), always be sure to contact your doctor *immediately*.

10. Antibiotics (except in very special problems such as certain heart infections or rheumatic fever) will *not* prevent secondary infections. In short, there is serious question about the prophylactic use of antibiotics, and you might well question the competence of any physician not familiar with this.

11. There are doctors who specialize in infectious diseases. These are the specialists particularly knowledgeable about antibiotics and the ones to turn to for help in an infection problem. Few in number, they are most often found in the university teaching hospitals.

And now for a unique drug-pusher.

11

Managing the
Medical Drug-Pushers:
Physician, Heal Thyself!

It's been said that the only thing greater than a patient's wish to have a magician for a physician is that physician's own desire to be a magician. With World War II those two wishes were virtually fulfilled simultaneously, in two areas at any rate, by the medicinal and drug explosion that took place. Suddenly, with a stroke of the pen on his Rx pad or a quick injection, the physician could strike down pneumonia, stop syphilis in its tracks, cure formerly fatal diseases, or change his patient's mood from severe anxiety to pleasant relaxation.

Truly it was magic; but, as when Faust summoned the devil to his aid, there was a price to be paid. Only now are we beginning to recognize the true dimensions of that toll, one so great that it threatens not only every individual who seeks a doctor's help but our entire society.

The two drugs Dr. Stolley found most often prescribed in the mid-Atlantic county mentioned earlier were those that satisfied this desire for a magical power to cure and heal—the antibiotics (the "miracle drugs") and the psychoactive drugs.

Only by understanding more about mood-altering drugs can you protect yourself and your family from a problem that has psychiatrists, sociologists, and public health physicians deeply worried. If we take Dr. Stolley's figure that 17 per cent of all Rx are issued for mood-altering drugs, and the total number of prescriptions dispensed in 1970 was over 2 billion, we find physicians must have written some 350 million Rx for psychotropic medications that year. Then there are the OTC psychoactive drugs bought as tranquilizers, sedatives, sleep aids, pep-up pills, or whatever. In 1971 (according to the reliable *Handbook of Non-Prescription Drugs,* 1973 ed.), Americans spent almost $29 million on over 100 different products to find better ways of getting to sleep and new ways of relaxing.

To cope with this avalanche of mood-altering drugs, to manage your doctor with his ever-present prescription pad, you must have the necessary information.

How Did All This Come About?

World War II sparked vast societal changes, put the world under the constant threat of the atomic bomb, and, since change always brings anxiety, produced a world that lives in fear. At the same time there was a vast technological leap forward. Not surprisingly, medical science benefited, and one result was the post-war discovery of psychoactive drugs—chemicals that could change moods, relieve the anxieties and depressions of man.

At the same time there developed a new, more efficient utilization of the media, particularly television, for advertising. With the favorable situation created by miracle drugs and their earlier promise, both professionals and laymen were prepared to accept advertisers' promises of chemical miracles with very little skepticism.

The result: a society in which consumers (and many professionals, as we shall see) feel that a pill should be the solution to all the problems that arise in the hassle of daily living, that drugs are a panacea for all man's ills. As our society grows more complicated, it produces more and more anxiety-producing problems. The pace of change has become too rapid for man to adjust to, as he did to the relatively slow changes of the past.

This situation was made to order for the pharmaceutical companies. They took advantage of it to advertise the mood drugs, both OTC and Rx, on TV and in the news media, as well as in medical, dental, and psychiatric journals. Knowledgeable sources estimate that several years ago the pharmaceutical houses were already spending $75 million on promotion annually—some $4,000 for each physician in the United States. This kind of money influences physicians through ads, gimmicks, and outright bribes (free samples of drugs, free meals provided at medical society or hospital staff meetings, etc.).

Out of this has come the attitude that we must not suffer any sort of mental anguish for even the most fleeting moment, that we mustn't be "blue," or fail to fall asleep within minutes of hitting the pillow, or fail to sleep uninterruptedly for at least eight hours thereafter. Any departure from such "perfection" must immediately be treated with mood drugs to achieve a Nirvana of the emotions, a super-health of the mind, if you will. As Dr. Robert Seidenberg, professor of psychiatry at the State University of New York at Syracuse, put it: "As a cigarette commercial once told us to 'reach for a "Lucky" instead of a sweet,' we are now in effect told to 'reach for a pill' instead of a thought!"

Why has the medical profession abetted this drug dependence, helped in fact to make it worse by reaching for a prescription pad instead of taking a few minutes to show real interest in a patient? Why have doctors rushed to prescribe instead of warning us against the OTC mood drugs? Why haven't they given us the help that can cure, instead of the drugs that only bury problems, making the patient worse?

The Physician Must Heal Himself First

A physician with cancer can treat a patient with the same disease; a practitioner with a kidney condition can treat a fellow sufferer. But the deviant physician (one whose behavior goes past the limits of propriety, the accepted norms of society) can help no one. The emotionally disturbed, alcoholic, or addicted practitioner can't be trusted to treat patients. Given the state of the profession, it's up to *you* to protect yourself and your family from these problems when you seek health care.

It's long been an open secret among those who've had an opportunity to see doctors in their off-duty moments that these medical healers are, as a group, in much worse shape than their patients. One might say that narcotic addiction, alcoholism, marital difficulties, and suicide are occupational hazards of the practice of medicine.

The incidence of narcotic addiction among doctors runs anywhere from 30 to 100 times that found in the population at large. Reports from the United States, England, Holland, France, and Germany indicate that about 15 per cent of the known drug addicts are physicians, although doctors make up just over one-tenth of 1 per cent of the United States population.

Dr. Ray L. Casterline, former president of the Federation of State Medical Boards and member of the Oregon Board of Medical Examiners, is widely respected for his knowledge of medical education. Recently he pointed out that each year suicide, narcotic addiction, and alcoholism wipe out a number of doctors equivalent to the entire output of seven of our medical schools: an average of 100 physicians are lost annually by suicide, 200 or more by narcotic addiction, and 400 or more by alcoholism.

Over a fourteen-year period Dr. Casterline has helped rehabilitate a considerable number of deviant doctors and has noted similar personalities and characteristics among them. His observations may help you in selecting your physician.

What to Beware of in a Doctor

Dr. Casterline has noted certain "pertinent identifiable personality factors" that he found common in most deviant physicians, regardless of how this deviance showed itself (alcoholism, drug addiction, suicide, etc.). He found in such doctors a chronic, needless failure to attend hospital medical staff and medical society meetings, a regular inability to complete patients' hospital records, and similar irresponsible behavior.

Think back for a moment to how we located a family doctor, and you see how our guidelines would eliminate the deviant physician. If your present doctor develops signs of irresponsibility, quiet checking may protect you from serious problems. Another good test is his marriage—unhappy personal relationships also form part of the pattern of the disturbed doctor.

The greatest tragedy lies in the profession's own conspiracy of silence, its refusal to discipline or heal itself. For the sick physician, usually recognized by his colleagues, fails to get help in time for himself, and his patients go unprotected. It's almost impossible to remove a doctor from practice when he has serious emotional problems, and only in the last few years have two states (Florida and Texas) passed a "Sick Doctor Statute" to protect the public. But what of the drugs that are often involved?

What Are the Mood Drugs For?

Mood drugs are not for the average person. They are for the truly mentally ill, such as mental-hospital patients, who with the aid of these potentially toxic drugs can return to society while psychiatrists work with them. In the very ill, powerful tranquilizers and mood elevators can be of great value, when utilized by specialists.

Mood drugs can also help the normal person to cope with the occasional crisis that arises once in many years: when one has to deliver an important public address or receive a major award; or a few days before serious surgery. But this sort of use doesn't explain the hundreds of millions of prescriptions cranked out by family doctors all over the nation year after year.

Why Are Mood Drugs Being Prescribed?

We're back again to the unfortunate fact that all too often an Rx is the way for a doctor to end a visit satisfactorily for everybody. But prescribing a mood drug leaves unexplored the patient's real problem, which would take the busy doctor too long to discover since it often lies buried in the unconscious mind. Estimates are that anywhere from over half to more than three-quarters of patients who seek doctors' help do so for vague psychogenic (emotional and not physical) complaints: problems whose causes lie in the sufferer's life-style, his day-to-day emotional problems, his hassles and tensions, his deep-seated psychological disturbances.

Unwilling to cope with such disturbing concerns, afraid of a time-consuming avalanche of emotional problems, the physician would much rather talk of some vague "functional problem," as if this were a diagnosis and not a semantic screen to hide behind. To give legitimacy to this escape and to "do something," he writes an Rx for a tranquilizer. While the tranquilizers may cover some symptoms for the moment, the cause of the unhappiness is unchanged and will only come back to haunt the sufferer increasingly.

Are Mood Drugs Overprescribed?

Clearly the answer is "yes." Recently Professor David C. Lewis of Harvard Medical School surveyed doctors on whether they thought other physicians were overprescribing these drugs, and two-thirds felt they were. Well over half the druggists asked whether people were buying too many OTC mood drugs agreed that they were. This explains why in 1970 the drug industry turned out 5 billion doses of tranquilizers, 5 billion of barbiturates, and 3 billion of amphetamines.

The Dangers of Psychoactive Drugs

Quite apart from the possibility of the drug reactions, which occur with virtually all chemicals, mood drugs may put the patient on a chemical seesaw. Often a hypnotic or sedative (say, a barbiturate) taken at night leaves the person so groggy in the morning that he needs an amphetamine to get going. So it may continue all day—a sedative to calm him down, then a pep-up pill to get him moving again, always on a self-operated chemical treadmill. Besides the danger of possible drug dependence, these medications tend to undermine confidence in personal mastery over the problems of life and can even prevent the solution of one's real problems through psychotherapy. As Dr. Mitchell Rosenthal, widely known psychiatrist and director of New York City's Phoenix Houses, put it: "Treatment by drugs is substituted for treatment by people."

The person who's just suffered the loss of someone dear is all too often the victim of these mood drugs. The Rx for sedatives makes the bereaved person less of a problem to doctor, relatives, and friends—but the sufferer pays for this. By preventing normal grief, drugs prevent proper recovery, and much damage can occur in the future. Here, too, drugs are being used to circumvent life in its normal manifestations and prevent the growth so necessary for health.

Drug advertisements even tell doctors how to relieve the anxiety of the young girl going away to college for the first time, which is cheating the young woman of a particularly critical period of growth and could lead to stunting, even possible psychological illnesses later in life. Doctors are even urged by drug houses to prescribe tranquilizers for children in school!

Many experts feel that doctors are at least in part the cause of our current drug-addiction problem. Dr. Donald B. Louria, noted drug expert and professor of preventive medicine at the New Jersey College of Medicine and Dentistry, calls attention to Canadian studies showing that if a mother is a daily tranquilizer user, her child is ten times as likely to use opiates, five times as likely to use stimulants or LSD, as similar children whose mothers are not daily tranquilizer users.

The OTC Problem and You

Managing your health care in the area of mood drugs involves managing your own impulses as well as those of your doctor. On your drugstore shelves are medicines supposedly able to put you to sleep, to calm jangling nerves or relieve irritability, to wipe out tiredness and fatigue. The dangers of the mood drugs are even more serious in the OTC area, because you don't even have a doctor to tell you when to take them.

Dr. Charles C. Edwards, former commissioner of the FDA, has pointed out that all OTC mood drugs are made from a few basic chemicals and that "most of these drugs are essentially ineffective in the dosages used and do have recognized side effects." Three investigators found basic mood-drug agents no more effective than a sugar pill. But some do suppress one important phase of sleep, the REM, or rapid-eye-movement, phase. This causes an increase in REM sleep on subsequent nights, along with nightmares that may lead the user to think he needs a drug for quiet sleep, and so he ends up psychologically dependent on the drug.

OTC sedatives or relaxants often contain the same antihistamines as OTC sleep aids, and experts can't figure out what makes the manufacturer decide whether to label a product a sleep aid, a sedative, or a daytime relaxant. OTC pep pills and stimulants all have caffeine as their active agent—a cup or cup and a half of coffee would do as well!

You're best off without OTC mood drugs: they have all the drawbacks of Rx drugs without their true mood-altering qualities; nor are they safe, except for the caffeine ones. Moreover, the realm of the emotions is the last place for the amateur to dabble. It takes the real "pro," the psychiatrist, to know when you should have a powerful mood drug. But how can you protect yourself from their promiscuous medical overuse, and assure yourself of getting them only when necessary?

Managing Your Doctor's Rx Pad

As we've already seen, a doctor is likely to reach for a prescription pad faster and oftener than Matt Dillon ever reached for his gun on *Gunsmoke*. Asking for "something" for an ailment of any kind is virtually sure to bring an Rx. And if you're entangled with a doctor who's too busy or not interested in *you*, the visit is almost sure to be ended by an Rx hurriedly written to clear the way for the next victim of an over-busy practice. Given today's medical scene, you're much more likely to find yourself with a doctor who's technically competent than with one who has any personal interest in his patients. You'll just have to learn to defend yourself by managing your doctor and his Rx pad.

When you discuss your problems with your doctor, it's best to ask what's wrong, then listen. Telling a patient a problem is "functional" is merely a lazy doctor's way of avoiding a diagnosis. A physician who spends the necessary time with you should be able to tell whether your problem stems from anxiety, depression (often the loss of a loved one), inner conflicts, loss of job, or whatever. If he's not sure or has no idea, it's time for either another doctor or at least a consultation. Once he admits there is no physical disease, you must be prepared to press for a detailed explanation. "But, Doc, what *is* wrong?" And then be ready to accept what you're told, perhaps some emotional fact you really don't want to know (or you would have recognized it yourself). But use your doctor's knowledge, help, and advice. Often, talking a problem over frankly, openly, and fully (why you need your doctor's time and not his Rx pad) with a knowledgeable and interested doctor will correct an emotional problem.

When a physician tells you, as Jerry's did, "I worry about the physical problems; then, if I can't find anything, I worry about the psychological"—you've got the wrong doctor. A diagnosis of an emotional disorder should be as positive as one of a physical condition, and the doctor should keep both possibilities in mind as he examines you. If he looks for one only when he can't find the other, he's likely to miss both.

You must initiate your visit with an openness, a willingness, to be told what *is* wrong. If you come in with a preconception, the physician may not want to waste the time converting you and may simply hand you an Rx for a tranquilizer. But if you tell him succinctly what's bothering you and then conclude with "What's wrong? What do you advise?" the way is left open for him and he feels no pressure either way. If he still reaches for the Rx pad, fall back on the questioning outlined in Chapters 9 and 10.

A well-balanced doctor, with some warmth and understanding and enough of a commitment to his patients to give them the time they need, can handle many if not most of the emotional problems of his patients. But the physician can no more heal himself than you can. When Hugh was told his violent cramps were "functional" and a prescription was shoved at him, he asked, "But, if this is emotional, shouldn't it be handled by psychological techniques and not drugs? I understand that talking is the way, either with you or a psychiatrist." The doctor's answer was to pooh-pooh it all. "Not necessary, just take those pills and the pain'll be gone. Hold on to the prescription number and if it bothers you again, you can get a refill."

Hugh finally got an answer from another family doctor, an internist who took the time to talk about the basis of his complaint, then suggested that they wait and see what happened. The cramps disappeared, without drugs, and there was no need for psychotherapy beyond the discussion.

The doctor who sneers at any specialty is not the doctor for you, for each specialty—psychiatry, gynecology, or whatever—has its important medical uses, and there's something wrong with the physician who can't use them at an appropriate time. Hugh had been careful not to ask for "something to be done," so he knew the pills shoved at him were his doctor's fault and not the result of his own pressure. Moreover, Hugh showed one thing you must be prepared to face (it disturbs most people): that some psychotherapy might be useful or even needed.

Points to Remember

1. The two drugs for which you're most likely to get an Rx are the antibiotics and the psychoactive drugs. Mood drugs are even available on a druggist's shelves for OTC sales. Since drug companies pressure doctors into using their products, you've clearly got to fight to stay clear of them.

2. Mood drugs relieve symptoms but only bury problems. They don't cure anything. If you use them, you are buying today's comfort at the price of further and possibly much more extensive trouble tomorrow.

3. Doctors are particularly susceptible to alcoholism, narcotic addiction, and suicide. A disturbed doctor is not the one to whom you can take *your* troubles for proper medical care. A deviant physician follows certain patterns you can check—regular failures to complete hospital records, needlessly missing hospital staff and medical society meetings, and other irresponsible behavior. A nurse in the hospital or a colleague, or perhaps a pharmacist, would be aware of his problems. A broken marriage is also a suspect sign in a doctor.

4. The mood drugs have very little place in the medication of the average person, although they are valuable to psychiatrists for the mentally sick. For the ordinary person a tranquilizer might be useful for a once-every-year-or-two occasion (for example, before major surgery).

5. When your doctor uses a prescription for a tranquilizer or other mood drug as a way of cutting short your visit, be suspicious.

6. The great majority of visits to a doctor's office are for non-physical complaints. The doctor who talks vaguely of "functional problems" and prescribes tranquilizers is taking the lazy way out. He should spell out exactly what the problem is (how anxiety, depression, or whatever, is causing your trouble) and spend time with you trying to straighten it out.

7. Beware particularly of the doctor who gives you one medication to relax you and another to lift you up if the first gets you down. This is putting you on a chemical seesaw, which can only lead to disaster.

8. The emotions and experiences of daily living, the everyday anxieties and depressions, are the raw material out of which we

develop and grow as human beings. Stunt this growth with mood drugs and you are preparing the way for serious psychiatric problems later on.

9. OTC mood drugs are generally ineffective, often potentially dangerous, and not for the amateur to fool around with.

10. If your doctor talks of "functional problems," ask for a consultation with a specialist—or find yourself another family doctor.

11. Be sure not to ask the doctor to "do something"—or you're likely to end up with an unnecessary Rx. Instead, ask for his opinion. "What's wrong here, Doctor? What do you advise?" If he still wants to give you a prescription, ask the questions outlined in Chapters 9 and 10.

12. If your family doctor puts down psychiatry, get yourself another doctor. Your physician must be prepared to use psychiatry or any other medical specialty at the right time, and for the right person.

13. *You* must be open and prepared to accept what your doctor suggests, whether it's to sit and talk over what's really bothering you or to see a psychologist or psychiatrist.

Now for the busy world of the pills and the no-pills.

12
Painkillers, Placebos, and Physicians

The painkillers or analgesics, the placebos or sugar pills, and managing your doctor—far apart as these may seem, they are actually the three-in-one, the Holy Trinity, of medical practice. All medical care is essentially the treatment of pain (the painful head, the painful gall bladder, the painful muscle or bowel or back), so the control of pain is at the core of medicine. The placebo is a powerful weapon in the hands of a person who knows how to use it, and it's been used since before the dawn of history. Man's first known painting—on a cave wall in southern France—is a drawing of the medicine man of some twenty thousand years ago. Arrayed in what was clearly the operating gown of his day, he's shown dressed in the skin of an animal, with large antlers on his head and stripes of paint on his arms and legs.

The importance of being able to manage your doctor will never be more clear than when pain casts its terrifying shadow. True, you can cope with that occasional sore arm or tension headache. But what of Carl, who rushed to a doctor for help every time he suffered a headache or sore finger, certain he had cancer? Or the unfortunates who live out their lives in chronic pain that torments them night and day—the person with severe arthritis or one of the bizarre pains so unbearable they have been known to drive sufferers to suicide (the neuralgia called "tic douloureux," phantom limb pain, or the terrible cluster headaches).

The other side of the coin finds chronic pain sufferers who just don't have enough pathology (disease) to account for the pain that causes them to be bedridden or entirely non-functional for at least twenty-two hours every day. These are the people who readily become drug addicts when doctors rely on drugs and not on themselves, permitting these sufferers to deteriorate to a point of no return.

Only by understanding all this can you learn to manage your doctor and get the proper help for your pain. So let's begin with your first line of defense against pain.

Your Doctor

In *The Doctor, His Patient and the Illness,* British psychiatrist Dr. Michael Balint puts it well: "... by far the most frequently used drug in general practice was the doctor himself...." If you watch your next appointment with a doctor, you'll realize the truth of this, and why it is so essential to find a really good family doctor. How well any pill is going to work depends largely on the way the doctor gives it to you, what he expects from it, and what confidence he inspires in you. In short, the remarkable help that is given routinely in one doctor's office may not be forthcoming in another's—because the doctors themselves are different, not because they know any more or less, have magical instruments or strange devices.

This is another reason why the selection of a doctor is so important. Ask yourself: "Do I trust this doctor? Do I feel he's doing his best for me? Do I feel he knows what he's doing? Can I rely on his sincerity, honesty, and judgment, his concern for *my* welfare?" If you can't answer "yes" to all of these, find yourself another doctor. Here the drug "doctor" comes in, for two men may actually be equally competent, interested, and sincere, yet communicate differently. For unconscious reasons you may not be comfortable or happy with Dr. A., while Dr. B. is perfect for you. Trust your feelings. Right or wrong, these will determine the way the drug "doctor" is going to work on you.

The Painkillers (Analgesics)

Americans probably consume more analgesics than any other single class of drugs. In addition to the amounts of non-narcotic analgesics prescribed by doctors (these rank third in Dr. Stolley's survey of most commonly prescribed drugs, behind only antibiotics and tranquilizers), we must add the narcotics given by mouth and injection and the $600 million worth of oral analgesics purchased over the counter by the public in 1971. Actually, it's impossible to conceive of Americans suffering so much pain that they would really need this amount of analgesics.

Here, too, there must be an abuse of drugs. Again, the physician doesn't want to spend the time finding out what really hurts his patient—whether it's arthritis, a sore arm, or simply the painful emotions. It's quicker and less troublesome to get rid of the patient with the mutually satisfying act of writing out an Rx. The patient himself is in no position to sort out these factors objectively but may just go down to the drugstore and buy a bottle of some analgesic—aspirin or a compound or whatever.

Were physicians willing to take the time, they might find out the real problems. Mary, referred for "severe" facial pain after getting no relief from several doctors and dentists she visited, finally reached one who just sat and talked with her. The fear of a cancer such as her mother had soon came out—and this fear exaggerated the uncomfortable pressure from a new dental bridge and caused her severe facial pain. Once she had reassurance and understanding, the pain was no longer a problem. Actually, nothing was done for her except to relieve her anxiety and provide some insight.

Some 60 to 80 per cent of the complaints doctors see are emotional in origin. These could be treated without drugs, but they do need the time and understanding that Mary received. Moreover, once analgesics are tried and the real problem remains, the patient returns to the doctor without relief (no aspirin could help Mary's pain) but with more fears. The apparent failure of the medication reinforces the patient's fears of the disastrous nature of the problem. The doctor, recognizing that there is no disease present, begins to form a picture of the patient as a "crock," a nuisance who upsets his time schedules or—what's worse—refuses to cooperate by getting better.

As the doctor continues to fail with drugs, he feels increasingly helpless and angry, so he increases the dosages of drugs, making them stronger. Eventually (unless the patient has enough awareness to find himself another doctor) the patient is turned unknowingly into an addict by the addictive drugs the doctor uses.

Another ploy in this game is what one physician commented to a colleague at a staff conference: "If they keep complaining of their pain, and the analgesics and tranquilizers don't work, they must be crocks, so I advise them to see a psychiatrist. They likely won't go, but at least they're not likely to come to *me* again." Obviously, the psychiatric referral should have been made differently and not used as an attack, an insult. The need for psychiatric help should have been evident from the first visit; and the patient should have been referred out of concern for his welfare, not as a move in a battle between an "uncooperative" patient and a stubborn, unfeeling doctor.

How will the sensitive, concerned doctor treat such patients?

Placebos for You

Until very recent times most medication was placebo, with no real pharmacological action on the condition or disease for which it was used. The word "placebo" comes from the Latin "I shall please," and is used for medication given to satisfy a patient rather than for any real scientific efficacy. However, those prescribing placebos all too often fail to realize that the placebo, the sugar pill, actually and scientifically does work. It's just that it works in a different fashion from the conventional drug.

It's been proven scientifically that placebos can stop pain in 50 per cent and more of severe cases; across the board, placebos stop about one-third of all pain, even that of terminal cancer or following major severe surgery. So you may well respect the doctor who has enough medical expertise to use this entirely safe drug properly: few drugs in fact are more effective.

The placebo works only when the patient believes it's going to work: either because ads have convinced him or because he has confidence in the doctor who gave it to him (the mother's kiss of the child's hurt finger is a placebo). By wisely using sugar pills, the competent, knowledgeable doctor can keep drugs to a minimum and often control psychogenic pain effectively in those who cannot be helped or who will not accept psychotherapy. This is why you should leave the placebos to the doctors and limit your use of OTC analgesics to the occasional aspirin for a tension headache or a sore muscle after tennis, where the problem is self-limiting and your doctor has told you aspirin is safe for you.

Managing Your Doctor and the Pain Game

The big danger of chronic pain is the use to which it may be put and the way your doctor handles it. If you play the pain game, the pain becomes important as a means for you to gain ends important to you. You may get control of those around you, defeat the doctors by refusing to improve. Some people make a whole career of this game and become what Dr. Thomas Szasz, professor of psychiatry at State University of New York at Syracuse, called a "painful person."

In these circumstances many patients are turned into addicts by their own doctors, who prescribe ever stronger analgesics in their attempts to prove their worth, to "do something" as urged by patient, family, and friends. This can happen to any of us. But how do you prevent this happening to you?

Here you must manage your doctor with care and sensitivity, using him and the specialists so that you safely get the help you need. First, tell the truth about everything you feel. It's fairly quick and easy for the doctor to examine you and see there's no disease but either an emotional problem or just a normal life process, such as arthritis as you pass into your forties and fifties. But it takes time to explain the process, to help a person accept his aging, in light of the American emphasis on youth and its supposed perfection.

With patients waiting outside and his own feelings of aging probably haunting him already, the doctor would rather scribble out an Rx for an analgesic, satisfied that he's "doing something" and making the patient feel fulfilled as well. If you can't get a family doctor who's different (there were only 5,800 F.P.s in February 1974 and they're the only ones trained for this sort of comprehensive care), you'll have to make the most of what you have. Your doctor may be excellent at scientific medicine, but he may still lack the *art* of medicine, simply because it has been ignored since World War II brought really effective drugs and different approaches to practice. So assess your physician and handle him with care. Even though he's understanding and competent, he may still fall into the common errors of practice if you press him too hard—and all doctors push easily.

Ask what's wrong: "Is there any disease present that's causing my pain?" If you can, ask about what really's bothering you (your wife or job or children or what-have-you). If you don't get a detailed straight answer, repeat the question, perhaps a little more loudly, and make sure you understand the answer, because it's often in medical jargon (see Chapter 13 for more details). And then: "Doctor, do you think anything should be done, or is this simply something I have to live with?" If you're concerned, you can also reassure yourself by asking if the pain does any harm.

Pain, though, is actually not a disease; it's only a symptom. Unless it's so bad you can't sleep or eat or function because of it, it will do no harm. In fact, it's often valuable in that it keeps you from doing too much. Phrase all this carefully; make it clear that you're *not* asking for something to be done.

Try to be as unemotional and objective as you can so that you don't arouse your doctor's pride about being able to control all disease and pain—or you'll get yourself an unnecessary Rx. If he still gives you one, ask what it is. If necessary, keep pressing the point until you know exactly what you're getting and why (you'll never read the Rx writing—pharmacists have enough trouble with it). If he throws a Latin name at you or a long chemical term, make sure you know how to spell it (then you can look it up in one of the volumes listed in our last chapter). Ask about side effects. If he starts getting impatient or refuses to go into details, you've got the wrong doctor—he either doesn't know as much as he should about what he's prescribing (perhaps he just got its name from his detail man), or he doesn't want to spend even this little extra time with you and so can't really have the time for you at all.

Finally, ask if there are any other drugs that can accomplish the same thing, and whether *any* drug is really needed or whether you'll recover as surely and rapidly without anything. Sometimes an analgesic like aspirin is used to reduce inflammation (as in arthritis), and you should know this too. From these answers you can tell how much care your doctor is taking, how much thought he's giving to your problems, how well he knows what he's doing. As a result, you may gain more confidence in and respect for him. Questions can often lead to positive results as well.

The Specialist in Pain

If your doctor can't convince you that he knows what your pain is all about, if he can't give you help despite repeated honest attempts on *both* your parts (some patients won't follow instructions), don't get hooked on drugs. The doctor should be able to diagnose the cause of your pain and offer a rational plan for treatment. If there's any question in your mind, ask for a consultation with a specialist in the particular area—a rheumatologist for arthritis, a neurologist for neuralgia—or with one of the growing number of headache clinics or pain clinics. If your doctor feels the problem has an emotional or psychogenic basis, a psychiatric consultation may well be in order.

For the sufferer who gets no help and is taking increasing amounts of drugs, there are the new pain clinics. These are usually accustomed to handling all sorts of strange forms of pain; they are knowledgeable in both the physical and psychological problems involved. Some have even developed complex ways of treating patients so that in a matter of weeks people who for years have been limited to moving between bed and bathroom are walking, able to travel and resume active lives.

How can you find a pain clinic or a headache clinic? Your doctor should know them, but if he won't or can't help he shouldn't be your doctor. You can locate them by calling the nearest university teaching hospital (preferably) or the largest area hospital or medical center and asking for the name or address.

Points to Remember

1. Before you can get help for your pain, ask yourself: "Do I trust this doctor? Do I feel he's doing his best for me and knows what he's doing? Can I rely on his sincerity, honesty, judgment, his concern for my welfare?" If you can't say "yes," find yourself another doctor. Trust your feelings. Right or wrong, they will determine how successful he will be with your pain.

2. Unless your doctor is willing to give you the time to sit and talk, to find any emotional causes for your pain, he may only put you off with increasingly strong drugs that still won't work. Beware of the doctor who just keeps writing stronger prescriptions instead of looking deeper into *you*.

3. The doctor who wisely uses sugar pills may be the most expert in the *art* of medicine and may be trying to protect you from unnecessary drugs. The placebo is certainly the safest of drugs, and few are more powerful.

4. Some people learn to play the "pain game," often being turned into addicts by the doctor who doesn't recognize the real nature of their problem. Here lies the importance of the insightful physician, the one willing to give you enough time to talk and find out.

5. Always ask what's wrong, what's causing the pain, and (this is the hardest) whether it's due to what you fear the most. Double-check any medical jargon to be sure you really understand.

6. Ask whether *anything* should be done or should you just learn to live with the pain (which is only a symptom and not a disease—in fact, it's often protective). Make it clear you're not asking the doctor to do anything, only to find out what's wrong and what he advises.

7. If the doctor gives you an Rx, ask what it is, if there are side effects, any alternative drugs, whether *any* drug is really needed or whether you'll recover as well and quickly without anything. If he gets impatient or avoids these questions, you must wonder whether he really knows the medication or is just repeating something the detail man may have just told him.

8. If you do as the doctor advises and, despite honest attempts on both your parts, there is no improvement, and if he can't

provide an exact diagnosis and proper treatment plan (if there is any), you should ask for a consultation—and he should welcome it. Ideally, he should have suggested one as soon as it became clear he wasn't able to help.

9. There are clinics across the country that specialize in diagnosing and treating pain. These setups produce amazing results in returning patients to normal functioning lives.

10. Beware the doctor who is vague about your pain and keeps prescribing stronger medication without suggesting a consultation with an expert.

And now for some tricks in talking to your doctor, and some special problems.

PART III
Doctor Talk and What It Really Means to You

13

What Your Doctor Must Be Made to Say—and What You Should Never Omit

Your doctor is probably suffering a bad case of "future shock," for he is a transitional creature. Coming from a tradition that relied on the art of medicine, on the relationship with the patient, the psychological support and personal help, today's doctor suddenly finds himself in a profession that focuses its attention on technological know-how. Thanks to a system of medical education that emphasizes the specialist and the scientist, the new doctors have lost touch with the old personal intimacies. Gone is the "bedside manner," which suddenly seems beneath the dignity of this new medical scientist.

The technologists who have taken over the medical stage have completely forgotten, or even sneer at, the father of medicine. Some 2,500 years ago, Hippocrates knew that his beloved medicine was an art whose Holy Trinity was composed of the disease, the patient, and the doctor. The physician was but the servant of the art, fighting disease side by side with his patient.

Family practitioners are trained specifically to take over this traditional role, but since there are only 5,800 of them among America's 350,000 doctors your chance of finding one is slim, although young doctors are increasingly turning to this specialty. Today you'll still have to accept the burden of communication with your doctor, but at least you can be sure—if you've used our methods of finding a family doctor—that your physician is competent, scientifically and medically, although you will have to compensate for his weaknesses and problems.

What *Not* to Do and What *Not* to Ask!

First and most important: when your doctor tells you what's wrong and what he advises, *don't panic!* Everyone is frightened and tense when he has a medical problem. Unfortunately most physicians have too many problems of their own to recognize those of their patients. For this reason doctors themselves characteristically avoid medical care and traditionally make bad patients. One surgeon told me that, faced with the need for surgery, he cut short his surgeon's explanation with: "Don't tell me. You're the surgeon, do it your way."

Typically, there is a frightened, tense, anxious patient and an authoritarian physician. This setup makes it difficult for the patient to exert his commanding position—after all, the patient commands the purse strings; he can use this doctor or find another.

Take Jim. He saw an orthopedic surgeon who told him: "You've got an arthritis of your thumb joint. It's unstable, and we'll have to operate and fuse it. You can wear a gauntlet but . . ." Virtually nothing the doctor said penetrated Jim's dense emotional smokescreen after the sudden prospect of surgery. And in another city, Barbara was told by her doctor, "We'll give you diuretics for this leg swelling . . . ," before she lost contact. Neither surgeon nor doctor even noticed that his patient missed almost all of what was said.

Actually, it took a week for Jim to sort out the pieces and call back to discuss his problem—to find that with a gauntlet (a sort of brace covering thumb, hand, and wrist) he could at least postpone surgery. And Barbara, who knew that diuretics were used by people with heart failure, went to see an internist, who told her all she needed was elastic stockings. She had varicose veins, and the prescription would have thrown her metabolism way off for no reason at all (it would have taken her doctor more time to diagnose the problem than to write out a quickie Rx).

Doctors don't always consider the effect of what they say, and often they speak bluntly, leaving the patient stunned and missing half the information. Add to the normal tension of a doctor's visit the medical jargon physicians often deliberately use, mistakenly believing that a certain distance between patient and doctor strengthens his image as a figure of authority, and you have a formidable gap to bridge in doctor-patient communications.

Dr. Barbara M. Korsch, a professor of pediatrics at the University of Southern California School of Medicine, carried out a study at Los Angeles' famed Children's Hospital by taping the visits of 800 mothers with sick children to the pediatrics clinics. The pattern she found was common to all medical practice and can teach you some of the tricks you need in order to handle your doctor. Almost half the mothers left without getting a clear explanation of what had caused their child's illness, and nearly one-fifth didn't know what was wrong with the child. More than one-quarter of the mothers never got to mention their greatest concern to the doctor, and some were so anxious or panicky that they didn't listen to what the doctor said. Some of the longest visits were a waste of time, with doctor and mother trying to get on the same wave length and never quite succeeding.

More than half the time the doctors lapsed into medical jargon that was merely confusing. One mother thought a "lumbar puncture" (removing fluid from the spine) was an operation to drain the lungs, while "incubation period" was thought to be the time a child was to spend in bed. Told a child would have to be "admitted for a work-up" or that doctors would have to "explore," most mothers didn't realize that these terms meant, respectively, hospitalization or a surgical procedure.

Such confusion goes on all the time. Doctors ignore the way they present material to a frightened patient, talking medical jargon instead of simple English. They do not know how to get explanations across, or just do not want to spend the time needed for presenting information. If you expect to know consistently what's going on in your health care, you're just going to have to learn to handle your doctor.

If the doctor's news is sudden and shocking (say, surgery is needed), don't try to absorb it all at once; give yourself a few minutes and then ask the doctor to repeat slowly what he said so that you can be sure you didn't miss any important elements. Try to ask about each aspect. What is wrong with you? What he is proposing to do about it? Is there any alternative? How safe is it? Will there be any side effects or complications? Is it *the* procedure to be followed or is there some controversy about it? Move on to how long it will take, what can go wrong, and how often complications occur. Ask him to explain any words he used that you don't understand. If you're very shaken, it's good to take some notes so that you can refer to them later. And if you're really shaken up, make another appointment and come with someone who doesn't lose his or her head, preferably someone with some knowledge of the area. It might be well to have a session with your family doctor if this visit was with a specialist. A phone call to clear up some of the confusion beforehand might help, but best of all would be a session with your family doctor, who can interpret the specialist's advice.

Very often, misunderstandings lead to long days and weeks of suffering for no reason; medical jargon or inadequate communication can terrify a person into some completely mistaken thought. If the situation is very serious, have the details worked out and clearly understood. Before the second visit, use the reference works in our last chapter to clarify your mind and then go into more detailed books in the library. *Be an expert on your own problem*—then you can really find out in the second visit what's going on. Do all this checking before you get another consultation, so you can make the most out of the information given you, so *you* know what to ask.

Talking out your problems with a friend or relation can be invaluable, because something you didn't realize you knew may slip out and answer some of your questions.

"What Did He Say?"

What you think your doctor said is just as important as what he did say, because you'll act on what you heard, and misunderstood instructions can make treatment fail. It's important to get a doctor on your own wave length—or to learn to tune in on his. Always ask when you're not sure, because many doctors are particularly vague. "I want you to lose some weight" (one pound, five, twenty?) ... "Cut down on your fluids" (half as much water, tea, coffee, what?) ... "Don't work too hard" (work ten hours a day instead of your usual twelve, work only two days a week?) ... "Come back soon" (tomorrow, next week, next year?).

Learn to ask specifics—how many pounds, how much less, in how many days or weeks or months. You can seriously harm yourself by misinterpreting vague instructions. Ask!

How to Get the Most out of Your Doctor

Your doctor is no god, no superhuman blessed with omnipotence and eternal wisdom, always right and perfect, ever willing to sacrifice himself. In the psychological reality of the relationship, he is a father-image, a figure of authority, and when we are sick we become infantilized (regress to the role of a child), making the physician an even more formidable power figure.

But your doctor is just another human being, subject to the same need for motivation, gratification, and reward. If you want to get the most out of him, you had best think of giving him what he wants most—in effect, you must bribe him.

One of the best ways to motivate your doctor is simply to tell him that you have complete faith in him, you are putting yourself entirely in his hands. This emphasizes his sense of responsibility, which he usually has anyhow, and makes him want to try a little harder, be more available, perhaps give you a little more of his limited time. But don't try it as a ploy—most people can recognize phoniness. Do it when you really feel that way.

It also helps to pay your bills on time. If for some reason you can't, tell the doctor in advance, explain when you will be able to pay, and then do so, adding a note of thanks for his care and his consideration.

You Should Never Ask a Doctor "Why?"

When you ask a physician—or most people, for that matter—"Why did you do that?" you're likely to stir up feelings going back to childhood and implying: "Why, you naughty boy or girl, did you do that?" It's more likely to produce an unpleasant reaction than a simple detailed explanation. It's best to ask: "What will this medicine do for me?" or perhaps "What is this for?" rather than the potentially emotional "Why are you giving me this?"

Beware—Doctors Push Easily

It's easy to get the doctor to do what you want. Just the threat of losing a paying customer or the implication that the doctor down the street does a better job may make him do what he knows is wrong or unnecessary, simply because you want it. There are few doctors who can resist this sort of pressure.

And you will pay the price. Take Margaret. At forty years of age her Pap test showed cancer. She called the medical society and got the name of a gynecologist close by. She did no further checking, and she chose badly. She told him she'd heard that if the hysterectomy didn't include removing the ovaries the cancer could recur. Fearful of losing the case, he readily agreed to do both the hysterectomy and the removal of the ovaries. At forty Margaret went through her menopause and lost an important body organ that may protect women against heart attacks. A member of the family pressed to know the laboratory report: there was *no* cancer in the uterus (it had been removed entirely by the biopsy). What Margaret should have done, of course, was to find a gynecologist by the techniques we have described, and then she should have confirmed the diagnosis with a second consultation. She should have asked, "What do *you* advise?" instead of walking in and saying, "I want. . . ." Margaret has learned the price this costs.

Understanding the Doctor and the Specialist

To "be a doctor" is an amazing thing—it can't be learned like mathematics or shoemaking. It's something that either fits the person or doesn't; it takes a strange combination of guts, self-confidence, brazenness, and gall, what is called *chutzpah*. The doctor must be willing to take on the role society accords him—to prescribe powerful, even deadly, chemicals and drugs, to advise and perform assaults on the human body, to cut into the heart or brain or abdomen of another human being, to take a human life in his hands and by moment-to-moment decisions lose it or bring it through to health and safety.

To be a doctor means accepting the awesome responsibility of life and death. Some doctors can never do this and end up research medical scientists. Some lose their heads in the intoxicating wine of this power, forgetting that they have this role only because society gives it to them, and that they are no better than anyone else, only different.

But it is a hard role, and it takes a toll. Specialists who frequently deal with death, particularly surgeons, will often cut themselves off from all personal contact with their patients, freeing themselves to do what they must, without personal involvement.

However, with this type of doctor the patient suffers doubly, because he must go through a frightening experience without the help or support he has a right to expect. Here the role of the family doctor is highlighted, for he alone can take up the slack and fill it effectively.

Asking for Information

You have a right to know what's wrong and what's going on, but this may exact a price you must be willing to pay without complaint. You have the right to know, and increasingly hospitals and physicians will give you your medical records if you insist. But when you get them you have no right to say, as did one man: "My record showed I had cancer. You've ruined my whole life with this information, and I hold you responsible for the damage you've done by letting me see this!"

Before you ask to see your records or for full information, be sure you're ready to take whatever comes your way. You may be among those who *are* better off letting the doctor tell them as much as he feels they should know. But if you are sincere in asking and can act maturely, you will almost invariably be able to get the truth of your condition from your doctor.

What You Should Never Omit
in Talking to Your Doctor

When a doctor or nurse asks you how you feel, he is not just making small talk. Frank didn't want to seem silly by complaining of the pressure he felt in one eye, thought it must be his imagination, and so the brain tumor was missed at an early stage when it might have been curable. And Gus didn't want to be a complainer about his stomach ulcer and thought the nurse was making small talk when she wanted to know how he felt each morning. He kept cheerfully answering, "Just fine," until he ended up in emergency surgery when his ulcer perforated his stomach. *Always tell exactly how you feel*—good, bad, or indifferent—when doctors or nurses ask. They're not making routine chatter; they want to know for *your* sake.

Most of us tend to cover up when we feel we did something foolish or wrong. If you neglect to make an appointment as soon as you see blood in the urine or feel a breast lump or whatever, don't compound the error by concealing how long it's been there. *Always tell the truth.* This may make the difference between watching the condition or taking prompt action—and between life or death for you. Telling the truth includes everything from symptoms, to how faithfully you've carried out instructions on your sexual practices, to just about anything you can possibly be asked.

Always include the things that you may have noticed have changed: shortness of breath or pain; swelling or fever or bleeding; marked weight changes; hoarseness or coughing; nausea or jaundice; changes in bladder or bowel function; lumps or thickenings; any digestive changes such as indigestion, stomach gas, pain, or difficulty in swallowing; changes in moles or warts or other skin conditions; and any sores that don't heal. Of course, any of these that occur one day and are gone the next usually aren't very significant. What you should be concerned about are the ones that persist the next day and the day after that (by then it warrants at least a call to your doctor).

How Should You Present Your Complaints?

When the doctor sees a patient with a long written list of complaints his reaction is: "Oh, my God, not another of those!" He is likely not even to listen to that person, and so may well miss something important. Don't bother him with minor nonsense that you understand ("I had a cold that lasted ten days when it's usually gone in a week" . . . "My period was two days longer than usual this time"). Have your major complaints written out if you like, as I do, or at least well in mind, then go through them succinctly, describing each one (the significant ones: "This wart seems to be changing in color and size" . . . "I noticed bleeding in my urine the past few days").

If the doctor fails to touch on every complaint during his examination and discussion, repeat your complaint again, in a good loud voice if necessary, until it is clarified. Physicians are likely to be more interested in some strange medical fact they stumble on than in the aching shoulder that's really bothering you.

How to Ask for a Consultation

The best way is to be frank. If the problem is a serious one—a heart attack or a stroke, say—you want to be sure it's handled properly. No physician worth having will object to a patient's asking: "Would you mind if we had a consultation because I'd feel more comfortable?" Or simply: "Wouldn't a consultation be helpful in this?" Another approach might be: "I don't have any doubts about you, Doctor, but I'd just like to get another point of view." Or perhaps you might even blame it on the family—my wife, or husband, or mother, or daughter says, he . . . she . . . they . . . "would be happier with a second opinion, another point of view to be sure no stone has been left unturned."

A good doctor will welcome this for two reasons: if it's a serious condition a consultation divides the responsibility, and a doctor confident of his own competence knows a consultation will make the patient more trustful and improve the relationship.

What *Not* to Do or Say with Physicians

There's a story about the doctor who died and went to Heaven. He was infuriated that he, a doctor, had to wait on line with everyone else at the cafeteria. When he saw a white-bearded man in a white coat and stethoscope walk to the head of the line and get immediate service, he became intensely angry and stomped over to Saint Peter to demand an explanation. Peter whispered to him, "That was the Boss—he just likes to play doctor sometimes."

Many doctors forget that their role was granted them by society and that they aren't any better than the rest of us. But if you want the most from your doctor, don't puncture his little balloon. As a group, doctors like to play you-know-who, the all-good father, self-sacrificing, saving lives on every hand, above the grime of money and that whole bit. It's worth joining in the game to have his cooperation.

Medical ethics are meant to keep doctors from criticizing each other, so don't expect them to. Listen to what you're told when you get a consultation (the specialist is dependent on your doctor for referrals and his livelihood) and ask carefully phrased questions, not about your doctor, but "I've heard it said that. . . ." Then draw your own conclusions about your doctor's competence in handling your problem. Don't expect them from the specialist.

A Final Word on Prescriptions and Specialists

You've gone through all the procedures suggested in the last few chapters and are sure the Rx is safe and necessary. But always check to see that it doesn't conflict with the last one given you, if you're still taking it, and be sure that your doctor has it on your record (if he doesn't keep precise records, find another doctor).

Don't let the specialist dismiss you with an "I'll send your doctor the report." Insist that he discuss the matter with *you*. It's your body and your life, and you want to know what's going on with it. This comment may be a cover-up for your doctor's mistakes or just an attempt at the outward form of medical ethics. It's fine that the report will be sent on to your doctor (you can discuss it with him if you want to, and it's part of your permanent record), but the specialist should tell you the whole story so you can get any questions answered and understand the whole matter free of any distortions that your own doctor may introduce into the picture. It also permits you to double-check on your own doctor and be more sure of him.

Points to Remember

1. As Hippocrates knew 2,500 years ago, the art of medicine is composed of the disease, the patient, and the doctor. *You* are just as important to successful medical care as your doctor is. You must learn to do your part.

2. *Don't panic!* If tension obscures what your doctor said, go over the story with him then and on a second visit if need be. Get it all straight.

3. Learn all about your problem from books. Then visit the doctor or specialist again, even bring a friend or relative to pin down the medical jargon. Make sure you understand everything so you know what to ask.

4. Be sure you know exactly what your doctor said, for if you fail to carry out instructions properly you may do yourself harm. When a doctor uses such vague words as "often" or "many" or "soon" or "cut down," find out what he means in actual figures.

5. Your doctor likes to know that you're putting yourself entirely in his hands and then he'll try harder, feel more responsible. He also likes to get paid promptly; if something will hold you up on payment, tell him so and send him a check as soon as possible.

6. Never ask a doctor "Why?" Phrase the question without the "why"; it avoids a lot of potential problems.

7. Doctors push easily. It's easy to get one to do what you want but it won't be his best judgment. Why go to him if you don't allow him to do his best? If you can't trust him and follow his advice, you shouldn't be going to him at all.

8. You have a right to know what's going on, to see your medical and hospital records, but be prepared to pay the price, because you will have to live with that knowledge. If you don't feel you can, should it be very bad, let the doctor tell you whatever he thinks he should.

9. What you should *never* fail to tell a doctor: the whole truth about how you feel. Some important symptoms or signs are shortness of breath, pain, swelling, fever, bleeding, weight changes, hoarseness or coughing, nausea, jaundice, changes in bladder or bowel function, lumps, digestive changes, changes in moles or warts or skin, sores that don't heal. In short, any change that

persists more than a day or two warrants at least a call to your doctor.

10. Be succinct and present only meaningful problems. If the doctor misses something you asked, repeat it loudly and clearly until he pays attention.

11. Certainly no doctor worth having will object if you ask for a consultation in a manner that doesn't insult his abilities: "Wouldn't a consultation be helpful?" ... "I'd feel more comfortable with a consultation."

12. Don't criticize the medical profession or another doctor (even when fully justified) to your doctor. He can't take it, and you may lose his cooperation.

13. If your doctor gives you an Rx and you're already taking one, make sure he's reminded of this and that the details are on your medical record (if he doesn't keep precise records, look for another doctor).

14. Insist that your specialist discuss what's wrong with *you*. Don't let him say, "I'll send a report to your doctor"—he may be covering up for your physician. It's your body and your life; you have the right to know. It may also give you a further check on how much your own doctor really knew. There is usually no problem with this, and the report to your doctor is good because you can also discuss it with him and it's part of your permanent record.

Certain groups have specific problems in getting medical help, and now we turn to these.

14

Is There a Doctor in the House— for the Gay People, the Women, the Elderly, the Teenagers?

The medical profession, plagued by a rampant overgrowth of specialists and the disappearance of family doctors, has permitted certain groups to fall between chairs, to be cared for inadequately by today's virtually vanished G.P. Our current spectrum of specialists can't meet the needs of these four groups of Americans, who typify in many ways the plight of our minorities. Hopefully, the growing numbers of F.P.s will solve the problems, but an adequate number of these is still far off in the future. Meantime, the gay people, the women, the aged, and the teenagers with their special needs for health care are waiting in the wings.

Who Shall Doctor the Gay Person?

The homosexual, just like the heterosexual, has his health problems, ranging from the common cold to cancer, from stomach ulcers to broken legs, from heart attacks to anything else. Historically, the role of the homosexual has varied with the society and the times—from the ancient Greeks, who accepted homosexuality as normal, to societies that threatened homosexuals with the death penalty. Some primitive peoples regarded the homosexual as a person having magical powers.

For the gay person the problem is obtaining medical care in our time and place. Vast changes have taken place during the lifetime of many of us. One older physician recalls a medical text of the 1920s that classified the homosexual as a "psychopathic inferior." In 1974 the American Psychiatric Association voted to remove the term "homosexuality" from the *Diagnostic and Statistical Manual of Mental Disorders*. Still, the homosexual physician fears his own profession's condemnation and feels he must conceal his identity to protect his livelihood. This chapter is primarily concerned with the non-medical gay person, his special medical and health problems, and how he should handle his doctor to get the care we all need.

At the June 1973 annual meeting of the prestigious American Orthopsychiatric Association, Dr. Eugene E. Levitt and Dr. Albert D. Klassen, Jr., of the Psychiatric Department of the Institute for Sex Research of Indiana University, offered the first results of a national survey on sexual behavior and attitudes. Homosexuality produced the greatest disapproval, with nearly four out of five people regarding it as wrong, and three out of five feeling there should be a law against it. But America seems out of step with its own times, for more than one out of four advocated a law against sexual intercourse between unmarried adults, and more than half were for a law against adultery!

It was only in October 1973, through the daring of a courageous physician, that the presence of gay doctors was finally revealed. Thus began a new dimension in the understanding of homosexuality, allowing exploration of the problems of both homosexual doctor and gay patient. Dr. Howard J. Brown is a far cry from the stereotype of the effeminate, ineffectual, and rather obvious homosexual. He holds two professorships at New York University (in its schools of medicine and of public administration), besides having successfully filled roles as chief of New York City's Health Services Administration and administrator of New York's Health Insurance Plan. As a result he knows some 3,000 or 4,000 physicians in New York City alone and is probably the most knowledgeable one to speak on the difficulties of homosexuals—male and female—in obtaining health care.

Most problems arise from the attitudes and limited knowledge of the heterosexual physician about the homosexual person. Dr. Brown feels that most gay people are right in their belief that they will find neither sympathy nor tolerance among the great majority of straight physicians. "But we don't really know a lot of the things people would like to know, because homosexual patients don't identify themselves as homosexuals, and homosexual doctors don't either. In fact, I don't know of any practicing physician in this or any other city who openly acknowledges himself as homosexual. In the large cities, some are known because they have a very large homosexual practice—but if in these circumstances the doctor is asked publicly, he would deny or evade the issue."

Special Health-Care Problems
of the Gay Man or Woman

Dr. Brown advises most homosexuals: "Seek a homosexual physician if at all possible." How do you find one? Dr. Brown points out that you really can't know except through the "grapevine," or perhaps by the fact that a particular doctor has an almost exclusively gay practice. Such physicians do exist in the large cities—New York, San Francisco, Los Angeles, London, and the like. Otherwise there is virtually no way Dr. Brown knows of finding a doctor who would be particularly sympathetic, although the younger physicians are more likely to be tolerant.

Under most circumstances, Dr. Brown sees no reason for the gay person to tell the straight doctor about his sexuality. However, if the male homosexual has a straight physician, there are some circumstances under which self-protection demands that he do so. For example, if there's a question of venereal disease, the patient might well ask the doctor if he's had experience with this problem, because it isn't well described in the textbooks. As Dr. Brown puts it: "Many heterosexual physicians know very little about venereal disease in homosexuals." For one thing, the oral and anal manifestations of V.D. are less common in heterosexuals. But there are many diseases other than V.D. in which adjustments to a disease call for changes in a person's life-style, alterations that necessarily affect one's partner. Other diseases may call for the doctor's dealing with the sexual partner—in effect, the homosexual family.

Since Dr. Brown's courageous announcement he has received letters from female homosexuals explaining the problems they have encountered with gynecologists. One, for example, finally told her gynecologist of her sexual orientation because he kept pushing contraceptive pills at her. In fact, gay women seem to have a great many problems in getting understanding from their gynecologists. So serious is the problem of the lesbian pregnant woman that Dr. Brown even knows of one center which is now thinking of setting up a special counseling service for these women. So serious in fact is the over-all problem that one medical magazine—the respected *Medical World News*—in its January 25, 1974, issue, reported on a young woman in medical school whose sister lesbians anxiously await the completion of her studies so she can become their family doctor.

Are Gay Doctors Safe?

This question invariably lies behind the thinking of straight people who attack homosexual physicians, and particularly gay pediatricians. More perhaps than any other single accusation, this angers the homosexual doctor. Just like most of his heterosexual male or female counterparts, the gay physician is first of all a doctor, a professional. After all, we are not afraid that a female pediatrician or physician will take advantage of little boys (or grown ones either). And despite the widespread, confirmed stories of male physicians and psychotherapists who have sexual relations with their female patients, we don't think in these terms when we consider or look at the doctor, unless the particular individual does something to make us do so.

But myths and misbeliefs, particularly sexual ones, die hard, and only a realization of the large numbers of homosexual physicians can bring a sense of reality to this subject. The usual figures for homosexuality are some 4 per cent of the population (according to Kinsey) and as high as 10 per cent if we include bisexuals. So there are probably some 35,000 gay doctors in the United States —yet I have never heard or read of one molesting a child or adult. Moreover, the gay doctor is also likely to be more sympathetic toward women's liberation and its aims than the heterosexual physician with his close ties to the conservative standards of our society.

Who Shall Doctor the Woman Today?

There seems to be a good deal of intense anger at doctors among the women's lib people—"tremendous bitterness," as the very informative and useful book *Our Bodies, Ourselves* (by the Boston Women's Health Book Collective) puts it. The anger seems composed in part of a feeling that the attitude of the medical profession toward women is male chauvinism, and in part of a feeling that women are treated as children, addressed by their first names, that the doctor takes an authoritarian role (that of the father-image) to intimidate the woman. As we have seen, there is a great deal wrong with the medical profession, but the problem here is not male chauvinism, and some of the complaints are not a cause for concern.

The problems women complain of are simply those that the entire society faces—not male chauvinism, but the problems of the doctor himself. If you're to get the maximum from the doctor-patient relationship, you must accept the physician as a father-image so that he can play the role in which he's the most help to *you*. In this role, addressing a patient (male or female) by the first name is ordinarily a good technique for doctors to employ, for the patient's benefit. In this unique relationship, *all* patients are bound to feel somewhat intimidated. This is not a factor of sex but of the magical father relationship, which makes it so difficult for any patient to stand up to the doctor.

While a one-to-one democratic relationship is best, the more serious the situation ("Is it cancer?"), the more this unique father-image relationship can support and help you. If you have only a head cold, you can readily meet your doctor head on; but if you're faced with a life-threatening situation, you'll want every bit of support you can get. Moreover, this paternalistic relationship makes drug therapy more effective. So, rather than trying to tear it down, use it knowingly and deliberately to help your recovery, to provide the care you need. Regardless of the doctor's emotional problems and the things you dislike about him, you can use the techniques in this book to see to it that he does his job properly, and that's what really counts.

All the tricks we've discussed in choosing a family doctor or specialist also apply to the gynecologist, who shares the role of family doctor for the woman along with her internist (unless she has an F.P.). In choosing an obstetrician, you might want to ask his nurse, before making an appointment, how he feels about natural childbirth, so that you know he and you are on the same wave length. This way you can get the training you need and not run into a clash when it's nearly time for your delivery. You might also ascertain before your first visit whether he and his hospital will go along with you and your husband in your feelings about your husband's involvement in your labor and delivery.

On your first visit you should also clarify the question of anesthetics or analgesics during delivery. It's not wise to start with an obstetrician who disagrees strongly with you on these questions. Doctors tend to push easily, and you might force the obstetrician to do what you want. If this goes against his grain, you may be courting disaster. If you reach a mutual understanding in which neither one of you gives up basic beliefs, and medical circumstances require a change in plans, it's easier to accept on rational grounds without running into a serious emotional clash at the last minute.

The F.P. and the Woman

This is another area where the new F.P. may well fill an unmet need. Here is a doctor who will be interested in you personally (something you can't very well expect from today's specialists) and in your family as well. Those developing this new specialty expect that the F.P. will handle some 90 per cent of all your medical problems—among them what is called "safe obstetrics," which actually includes many if not most deliveries. It also provides a continuum of care, as the F.P. delivers the mother and then turns to care for the infant.

Selecting a Doctor for the Elderly

The majority of physicians are uncomfortable with the aged, and so are inadequate in caring for them. To find a doctor for anyone past sixty years of age is a major problem. This is a tragic area of neglected and unfulfilled needs with a very limited number of qualified physicians, making managing the doctor a more difficult job here than in most areas. And all despite the fact that one in every ten Americans is sixty-five or older—some 22 million aged (if you accept sixty-five as the arbitrary chronological cut-off point between middle and old age). More important than the reality—that any such arbitrary age is meaningless—is the societal myth, with its implied threat of physical and mental incompetence due to old age and the very real fear of impending dissolution. All of us, doctor and patient alike, are affected personally by the awareness of oncoming "old age."

This inherent psychological threat and the fear it arouses make the choice of a doctor depend in considerable part on the doctor's age. First, the physician should like the elderly person—if he's uncomfortable or dislikes the aged, or if he's patronizing, start. looking for another doctor. The best physician for the elderly is either the young man up to forty or so or the older doctor in his seventies. The very young don't feel threatened yet by age, nor do they identify with the patient or his problems; while the man past seventy has come through the storm and reached some sort of peace with himself and his age.

The in-between ones, doctors in their forties, fifties, and sixties, will identify with elderly patients and want to avoid them. Even psychiatrists (supposedly with better insights) are no exception. At a recent major national psychiatric conference two lectures were given simultaneously in different halls—one on adolescent psychiatry, one on geriatric (that of the aged). The adolescent session had the psychiatrists virtually hanging from the chandeliers, while the geriatric session had only a scattered few attending. This pattern happens consistently at medical meetings.

With this built-in resistance in the medical profession, which has failed so notably in other instances to heal itself, it's not surprising that the specialty of geriatrics is largely unrecognized and that formal post-graduate training is almost impossible to obtain except in a few scattered spots across our land. So obsessed with youth is our society that it's willing to write off one in ten of its citizens.

What the Doctor of the Elderly Must Be Like

Apart from the general age question already covered, this doctor must be a knowledgeable physician in the broadest sense. He must understand and appreciate how closely the elderly person is interrelated with the world about him, with his past, and with his childhood training of some fifty or seventy-five years ago. In short, he must look to the whole person and not the symptoms. But *most of all* there must be a certainty that the doctor is really concerned about the patient.

For one thing, the doctor who pulls a patronizing "isn't he cute" routine, who gets familiar on a first-name basis or calls the elderly person "Mom," "Pop," "Granpa"—this is not your man. This approach simply detracts from the elderly person's dignity and helps to tear down self-esteem, which is all too often at a low level because of our society's attitudes. As for the physician who tells an adult son or daughter, "What do you expect, he's an old man"—well, you've got an inadequate doctor who, faced with a situation he can't handle, falls back on the tragically derogatory stereotypes of the elderly too long perpetuated.

Care of the aged is a team approach more than any other area of health care. There is, for example, the home-care team: the doctor, the homemaker and social worker, the visiting nurse, physical and occupational therapists, the dentist, and the "friendly visitor." Vital to this team and often central to the entire life of the older person is the minister, who can be an excellent source of referral to a physician interested in the aged, for community programs and resources of value.

Finding a doctor is difficult because the specialty of geriatrics is poorly organized and meagerly staffed, and its practitioners hard to find. Asking a physician may not even help, because many are only minimally aware of such resources and have no personal contacts. Nor is a call to a medical school likely to be of much help, because the crowded school curriculum gives little recognition to the problems of the aged. The hope is that the F.P. will provide help here too.

There is another source of referrals, but it's tricky and often hard to evaluate. High-quality nursing homes, particularly those attached to large charitable organizations, have medical staffs whose doctors usually are interested in the elderly—but it's hard to evaluate these nursing homes, and very few are worthwhile. A call to a university teaching hospital may reach the right person, who will track down the right doctor. Certainly one of the nurses at a first-rate nursing home can tell which doctor seems most knowledgeable and interested. Rehabilitation institutions connected with university teaching hospitals are another source.

A Doctor for the Teenager: Ephebiatrics

Hebiatrics or ephebiatrics is the latest medical specialty. Before 1951 it didn't exist. That year the first unit was founded, in Boston Children's Hospital Center. Often called adolescent medicine, this sub-specialty of pediatrics has grown so rapidly that by 1970 three-quarters of our hospitals were interested in setting up adolescent services, with growing numbers of medical students getting training in such clinics. Adolescent medicine cares for the youngster too old for the pediatrician and too young for the internist, with a vague age range from twelve to twenty-one years.

With not many more adolescents than aged, our distorted society still gives more attention to the youth, who need far less and much simpler medical care. In fact, the F.P. can adequately provide a continuum of medical care for the adolescent, while the aged need a team approach.

In any case, adolescent medicine has come on like gangbusters, with new clinics and specialized training programs all over, active professional recognition, and doctors rushing into this "now" specialty. Like pediatrics, adolescent medicine involves the total care of the patient through a particular stage of life, whereas the classic specialties such as cardiology or dermatology or gynecology concentrate on the care of particular organs or organ systems.

Getting a specialist in adolescent medicine can follow the same pattern we described for finding a family doctor or specialist. Your internist or gynecologist may be able to recommend one, and you can check his qualifications just as you did those of your own doctor or specialist. Or you can call a medical school or university teaching hospital for the chief of staff or someone available in adolescent medicine, and then move down the line to the largest local hospitals and so on.

With the situation what it is, there will clearly be changes in the next few years, with official specialty recognition coming from the medical profession and board certification probably right around the corner.

Unfortunately, though, only public pressure will move the medical profession to put more into that rapidly growing segment of our population, the aged—very likely *the* most rapidly growing section, for the United States Census Bureau estimates that the number of citizens over sixty-five will increase by well over 50 per cent between 1960 and 1985, while our population growth seems to have come to a virtual halt.

15

How to Get Help
for Your Sexual Problems

As we've seen, your doctor is likely to be uptight and confused about many things. Bound by the life-style and conventions of the society from which he has sprung, he finds himself torn between comfortable tradition and the tensions of change. He still faithfully reflects our country's attitudes toward everything from homosexuality to possessions, from status to the use of prescriptions. His emotional problems are clearly greater than those of the people he treats—as evidenced in the higher rate among physicians of narcotic addiction, alcoholism, suicides, and broken marriages. So you really shouldn't be too surprised if you face difficulties when you turn to your doctor for sexual information or for help with the daily problems of human sexuality.

The best way to deal with this always touchy subject is to handle your doctor carefully, to feel your way, to test him to see how far you can raise sex questions with him. A slow, cautious approach will reveal how much he really knows about human sexuality, and what prejudices and problems he has, so you know how far to trust him.

The Real Problem

The real problem that doctor and patient together must face today is the sexual revolution that has burst upon all of us with the sudden fury of a summer shower. Ordinarily mankind has seen gradual changes over a matter of centuries, so that people had a chance to adjust, to develop new patterns, to find ways of coping with changed situations. But since World War II simultaneous social, intellectual, cultural, scientific, and technological explosions have blasted all our established patterns, leaving many of us floundering and trying to find some sense or meaning in this strange new world, while others can't appreciate or understand what went before and are only concerned about living "now."

Our fast-changing societal attitudes toward everything from abortion to the Pill, from V.D. to homosexuality, have taken a terrific toll of the doctor-patient relationship. Ours is a period of transition so traumatic that it's hard to see the present without trying to foretell the future.

This chapter offers you ways to manage your doctor so that you can get the latest in sexual information. It can help you find the doctor who can help you, and teach you how to protect yourself from the many self-styled medical experts prepared to tamper with the dynamics of human sexuality despite totally inadequate preparation.

Sexual Confusion and Doctor-Patient Relations

The doctor today is confused. He comes from a world in which patients rarely talked to him about sex—in fact, until very recently people rarely talked frankly to anyone about sex. Probably only the psychoanalysts did any real talking about sex until after World War II, and many psychiatrists are still not trained to do so adequately, according to today's experts in this relatively new field of human sexuality.

But today's family doctor is likely to find his most "respectable" and conservative patients suddenly talking to him of oral-genital or anal sex; of masturbation, homosexuality, and lesbianism; of sexual orgies, group sex, and wife-swapping; of fetishism, transsexualism, and transvestitism. He's likely to be asked about the advantages of certain sexual positions or for information on others. And certainly he will face much freer discussion of orgasms, premature ejaculations, and impotency. Only the young doctor who has recently graduated, who grew up with the sexual revolution, is likely to feel completely at home in this new atmosphere—unless the doctor learned long ago to be free inside himself, to incorporate new values and new attitudes, to accept change of the most radical sort.

But this new-found freedom, this sexual revolution, has in no way wiped out sexual problems or even reduced them. The most it's done is simply to change the mixture, adding new ones to the old. Venereal diseases, which had almost disappeared, are back in epidemic and often more virulent forms. Dr. René Dubos—famous bacteriologist and first to develop deliberately and prove an antibiotic—is certain that no antibiotic, old or new, will control this epidemic until social conditions change once more.

Which Family Doctor
Can Advise You on Sexuality?

This question must be approached in two ways. First, there's the family doctor you've had for some time (and who may not recall the original interview); second, there's the new doctor you're about to see and judge.

In general, there's an appalling lack of information on sex, for until the last few years doctors got little or no academic training in human sexuality. As recently as 1961, only three medical schools in the entire United States offered courses in human sexuality. Today, however, courses in this field are being given in many medical schools and their numbers are increasing. Your problem in finding a doctor in this area is that only some of the doctors who've graduated from medical school within the past decade have had academic training in this field, and these have had so little experience that you might well hesitate to use one as your family doctor.

But regardless of the training these young doctors got in the anatomy, psychology, and physiology of human sexual behavior, the way the practitioner handles sexual problems essentially depends on how he can or cannot handle his own sexual hang-ups. For this you have to depend on your own insight, and on managing your doctor.

Sexual taboos have existed since man first emerged on this planet and have pervaded every society and culture. They have varied from avoiding the menstruating woman as "unclean," to prohibiting athletes from masturbating or having sexual intercourse the night or day before a big game. The Puritans prohibited sex on Sundays. Now intercourse is generally permitted except in special cases after heart attacks—although the heart rate can go up during sex from the normal 70 beats a minute to 150, while the blood pressure rises from 120 to 250 and more. There's the old story of the doctor who told a patient who'd had a heart attack that it was all right to have sex, "but only with your wife, I don't want you to get excited." Strangely enough, there may be something in this old wives' tale: a recent study of men who died of heart attacks as a result of sex revealed that 27 of the 34 actually were having extramarital relations.

Hopefully your doctor has had some background in human sexuality and is free of the myths and taboos so common in our society. If the doctor is new to you, the first visit will be your physical examination and should include a careful medical history. Here will be your basic tip-off on your doctor's aptitudes and attitudes in the field of human sexuality, for he should find a way to lead you into a careful and detailed sexual history just as comfortably as he does with your medical history. Some doctors start with a simple question about present or former marriages. From that point, a good doctor will go subtly, feeling his way along, moving on as you relax and respond to increasingly probing questions. He will go as far as any anxiety of yours will permit; he may use a prepared or printed questionnaire or just talk. He'll check frequency of intercourse, your feelings about it, impotency and frigidity, orgasms, premature ejaculations, sexual positions and techniques, just about everything likely to play a role in your sexual life.

But while he's checking you out, you can be checking him as well! He should be comfortable with his own questioning. If he's ill at ease or seems awkward, if he falls back on technical or scientific terms rather than the usual sex words we all know, you can be suspicious of his ability to deal with his own sexual hang-ups. He should make you feel he's accepting and tolerant of all attitudes and feelings, that he's honest and not going to pass judgment on your actions or beliefs but give them acceptance and respect. He should be sensitive to your feelings and reactions, sincerely interested in *you*, and have no personal embarrassment at whatever sexual material you bring up for discussion.

It's a big order, but if the doctor can't fill it he shouldn't try—his hang-ups will only make yours worse. If your doctor isn't capable of fulfilling his role in sexuality, you have a problem whose resolution depends on why you went to this doctor in the first place. If you just go for a routine physical check-up and the doctor is all right otherwise, you can sit tight and ask for a referral should a sexual matter later arise. But if you go to the doctor because you have a sexual problem, it is immediate action that you need, and if he has too many problems to take an adequate sexual history, you're not likely to get any help in this area. In that case you have to seek another family doctor or ask for a referral promptly.

The real difficulty arises when you have a hidden sexual problem—vague pelvic pains, exhaustion, fatigue, difficulty in concentrating. A doctor who is uncomfortable with sex is not likely to want to diagnose sexual problems and might put you through extended tests looking for a non-sexual cause for a sexual problem. Here you must be alert enough to suspect the possibility of a sexual basis for vague, ill-defined problems and ask for a consultation or see another family doctor promptly.

If you've had a family doctor for some time, the pattern works a little differently. Say you open the discussion with "Doc, I can't get it up like I used to," or "I'm unhappy, I read so much about other women with their climaxes and I can't seem to have one." From his reaction you'll know immediately how well your doctor can handle sexual problems. If he then sits down and takes a careful, competent sexual history, the first hurdle is over.

But if your complaints are the vague ones of an underlying sexual problem he may either do the same, in which case you can relax for the moment, or he may get involved with a long series of tests. In that case you might ask, "Doc, is there a possibility this may be a symptom of a sexual problem?" And if you get an embarrassed or a pooh-pooh sort of vague answer, you know it's time to look for either a referral or another family doctor.

What Can You Expect from a Family Doctor?

The family doctor is probably the first port of call and can be quite successful in many sexual problems, if he's as knowledgeable as he should be. As Dr. Warren J. Gadpaille, an Englewood, Colorado, psychoanalyst and nationally known expert on human sexuality, has pointed out, the vast majority of patients the family doctor is likely to see are not the more bizarre problems such as fetishism or transvestitism, but men beginning to have problems with potency and women who are not orgastic and whose reading has left them newly dissatisfied.

In the simpler sort of problem, often all that's necessary is reassurance, for many times the problem is simply a passing occurrence. As Dr. Gadpaille has pointed out, frequently a man who doesn't drink much goes out and gets plastered; he comes home to make love to his wife and is impotent for the first time, and it scares him. He waits a few days to get over the fear and decides to try again. To get up his courage he has a few drinks, and he's impotent all over again. He goes to his doctor, who reassures him: "Look, it's nothing. Just don't drink any more before you have sex." The problem is solved; the man is happy and potent again.

According to Dr. Gadpaille, there is a whole series of drugs which can cut down sexual potency: many tranquilizers, for example, and some of the drugs patients take for heart conditions. A knowledgeable doctor recognizes the reason for this impotency and says, "Let's see if we can't find a drug for you which will give the desired physical effect without this sexual problem."

Dr. Gadpaille feels that taking a careful sexual history is the best proof of the qualifications of your gynecologist. While women are getting less afraid to talk about sex, they still need more encouragement than men. Gynecologists, accustomed to female sexuality, are more capable of handling it than the family doctor, and they aren't as scared by it. But what of the qualifications of the family doctor or psychiatrist who offers sexual help?

How to Check the Sexual Counseling of Family Doctors and Psychiatrists

You cannot assume that because your family doctor can take a good sexual history he can also deal with complex problems. Unfortunately, some doctors seem to think reading a couple of books (Masters and Johnson, perhaps) and attending a few lectures and maybe a half-day seminar are sufficient qualifications. Let's see what happens and how the patient can handle the situation to protect himself.

The patient comes in and the doctor asks about his sex life. With a sigh of relief the patient unburdens himself. He and his wife are having troubles—she's not very orgastic, he's bothered by premature ejaculations. The doctor says, "Oh, we can help that." At this point the patient should ask the physician in a friendly way, "Doc, I've naturally been reading up on this, and my impression is that people who can really work with these problems are the ones who handle it almost like a sub-specialty—the doctors who've gone to St. Louis and spent six months with Masters and Johnson, gone through the program out there to learn how to use these kinds of therapies, or worked with other leaders in this field. They really have to devote a good part of their time to this field. Has this been part of your special interest? Did you work with Masters and Johnson?"

The physician who gets annoyed by such a question, or who fails to answer with full details on his special training in this field, may well have something to hide. If you don't get detailed evidence of proper training in human sexuality, it's time to look for another doctor. If you're starting with sex problems, an untrained or inexperienced practitioner will likely only make matters worse and leave you with more problems than before.

Psychiatrists, too, may not be qualified to handle sexuality— apart from the psychoanalysts (only about one in twenty psychiatrists is a practicing analyst), who are generally excellent in this field, according to Dr. Gadpaille. You might well ask the psychiatrist for his background as you did the family doctor, and also: "What do you think of such a problem [whatever yours may be]? Have you had experience with it? How successful have you been? What's your philosophy of treatment?" If the psychiatrist says the problem is hopeless, he's never had success with it, get another psychiatrist.

Seek and Ye Shall Find:
How Common Are Sexual Problems?

Many patients avoid discussing sexuality; their doctors usually have to work to bring out sexual problems, unless they are the reason for the visit. And because of the discomfort some doctors feel in this area, other patients tend to shield the physician from embarrassment, even when they themselves are quite willing to talk about it.

Surveys reveal that the number of sexual problems found is related to the doctor's comfort and ability with sexual histories. Those who handle the matter naturally and easily, who ask routinely about sexual problems, found some 15 per cent of their patients reporting sexual difficulties; while those who asked only when it seemed indicated found only half as much. Those doctors who showed distinct discomfort in discussing sex (blushed or fidgeted, became angry, obviously avoided sexual terms, or were uneasy in other ways) reported sexual problems in well under 3 per cent of their patients.

Any doctor who felt uneasy about taking a sexual history would react similarly if a patient brought up the subject of sex or its problems. The doctor would thus effectively choke off the presentation of any sexual problems by his patients—a way of protecting himself from those things which caused him anxiety. Most patients would pick up the doctor's discomfort in this area and immediately stop talking about it.

In its excellent volume *Human Sexuality*, the AMA and its Committee on Human Sexuality illustrate the dangers of asking the doctor with his own sex hang-ups about yours. A young wife saw her family doctor about a sexual problem. In the course of the consultation she asked what "fellatio" meant. The doctor explained and then remarked that only homosexuals and perverts used it. Until then the young couple had practiced and enjoyed fellatio, but the overwhelming guilt feelings that arose from what her doctor had termed "perversion" finally forced the young woman into psychiatric care.

It's obviously important to ascertain your doctor's feelings about sexuality before you entrust these deeply felt and sensitive areas of your personality to him. In our next chapter you will find listings for three excellent volumes that can offer you scientifically accepted advice by authorities in the field, and a competent physician or the AMA's Committee on Human Sexuality can suggest other material.

Points to Remember

1. Your family doctor is likely to be confused and disturbed by the sexual revolution he's living through, and he's probably had little or no training in handling sexual problems, so you have to find out his background.

2. If your doctor has had some training in human sexuality and has control over his own sexual hang-ups, you'll sense it in his approach to your medical history. If his questioning about the sexual aspect of your life is gentle and makes you feel at ease, it's a good sign that he is knowledgeable, and he may be able to give you a lot of help. If he's awkward and makes you feel uncomfortable about discussing sexual problems, forget him and ask for a specialist in the field.

3. You must learn to be alert to signs of sexual problems—vague, ill-defined problems with no definitive medical or physical findings.

4. Take nothing for granted about a family doctor or even a psychiatrist where sexual know-how is concerned. If he suggests any form of treatment, ask: "Have you had specialized training in human sexuality? Is it your special interest? Did you train with Masters and Johnson?"

5. Psychoanalysts in general have had good training in this field, but not *all* psychiatrists or psychologists. Ask if they've had success in handling others with *your* problems.

6. Don't talk sex to your physician until you've ascertained his ability to cope with the material or he can do damage. If you just feel he would be uncomfortable in this area, trust your own feelings—they're most likely to be right. Discuss this only with doctors you feel can handle it comfortably and who show signs of knowledge. Don't hesitate to ascertain their training before going ahead with any suggested therapy.

And now for some books that will be of use to you in your task of managing your doctor.

16
Your Home
Medical Library

Books That Will Help You to Manage Your Doctor

To cope with doctors, you must be prepared to check on the medical jargon, the terms, the vague comments they make, and this can be done only by accumulating a library of your own. Then there are other books which you should at least look over and become familiar with, so that you can use them if the occasion arises. Later you may want to buy some of these if you find you are comfortable with them and use them enough.

Let's start first with the basic books that you should own.

MEDICAL BOOKS FOR THE HOUSE

Brown, J.A.C., *The Stein and Day International Medical Encyclopedia.* New York: Stein and Day, 1972.

Clark, R.L., and Cumley, R.W. *Book of Health.* 3rd ed. New York: Van Nostrand-Reinhold Company, 1973.

Nourse, A.E. *Ladies' Home Journal Medical Guide.* New York: Harper and Row, 1973.

These books are excellent and authoritative, with broad coverage. The *Book of Health* is a little more scientific, perhaps, with more history, while the others may put slightly more emphasis on newer medical problems such as abortion. It's best to compare them in the bookstore or library before purchasing one, since they're not cheap.

Boston Women's Health Book Collective. *Our Bodies, Ourselves.* New York: Simon and Schuster, 1973.

Phibbs, B. *The Human Heart.* 2nd ed. St. Louis: C.V. Mosby, 1971.

These two are specialty books. *Our Bodies* is a wide-ranging book on the medical, social, personal, and sexual aspects of womanhood. *The Human Heart* is for the heart patient and his family, anyone interested in the heart in fact—completely authoritative.

American Medical Association, Committee on Human Sexuality. *Human Sexuality.* Chicago: AMA, 1972.

Everything you might want to know about every aspect of sex; completely authoritative; the excellent glossary and bibliography will prove invaluable.

Stedman's Medical Dictionary. 22nd ed. Baltimore: Williams and Wilkins, 1972.

Invaluable if you want to keep up with your doctor and his jargon.

Gomez, Joan. *Dictionary of Symptoms.* New York: Stein and Day, 1968.

A convenient guide to interpreting danger signals and symptoms. Tells what you might have, what you definitely do not have, when a doctor is needed.

BOOKS FOR THE MEDICAL DRUG SCENE

When you get an Rx thrown at you, or a friend urges some OTC medication, or your doctor throws some medical term at you, you can check the drug in one of the following volumes, all either useful in special areas or particularly authoritative or easily obtainable.

AMA Drug Evaluations (prepared by AMA Department of Drugs). 2nd ed. Acton, Mass.: Publishing Sciences Group, 1973.

An authoritative and very valuable volume on drugs and their uses and doses.

Handbook of Non-Prescription Drugs. 1973 ed. Washington, D.C.: American Pharmaceutical Association, 1973.

Authoritative coverage of the OTC market with considerable informative material and figures.

Physicians' Desk Reference (annual). Oradell, N.J.: Medical Economics, 1974.

Has photos so that you can identify virtually any tablet or capsule by size, shape, color, number, and so on.

Fisher, R.B., and Christie, G.A. *A Dictionary of Drugs.* New York: Schocken Books, 1972.

Limited in coverage but widely available.

Goodman, L.S., and Gilman, A. *The Pharmacologic Basis of Therapeutics*: 4th ed. New York: The Macmillan Company, 1970.

Authoritative and outstanding.

SOURCES ON SEXUAL PROBLEMS

McCary, J.L. *Sexual Myths and Fallacies.* New York: Van Nostrand-Reinhold Company, 1971.

Useful to put many of the old wives' tales to rest.

Masters, W.H., and Johnson, V.E. *Human Sexual Response.* Boston: Little, Brown and Company, 1966.

Need more be said?

MORE TECHNICAL MEDICAL AND PSYCHIATRIC VOLUMES

The Merck Manual. 12th ed. Rahway, N.J.: Merck & Company, 1972.

Relatively simple medical text and virtually a classic.

Solomon, P., and Patch, V.D. *Handbook of Psychiatry.* 2nd ed. Los Altos, Calif.: Lange Medical Publications, 1971.

A simple source book of psychiatric knowledge with an interesting chapter on doctor-patient relationship.

De Coursey, R.M. *The Human Organism.* 3rd ed. New York: McGraw-Hill, 1968.

Basic principles of human anatomy and physiology at the college level; easily understandable and authoritative.

Frank, J.D. *Persuasion and Healing*. Rev. ed. Baltimore: The Johns Hopkins Press, 1973.

An excellent consideration of the varieties of psychotherapies today.

Freese, A.S. *Pain*. New York: G.P. Putnam, 1974.

Detailed consideration on special areas of managing your doctor—the pain game, the pain doctors, misuse of drugs, placebos.

"Standards for Cardiopulmonary Resuscitation" (CPR), supplement to *JAMA*, February 18, 1974.

CPR—the whole story. *Important:* you can obtain a copy through your local Heart Association, or the American Heart Association, New York, N.Y. 10010.

In addition, many of the standard encyclopedias are excellent general sources of information.

CHECKING YOUR DOCTOR, DENTIST, AND HOSPITAL

In most sizable libraries you will find the volumes you need to check the background of professional people and hospitals. Your librarian is an invaluable source of help. If your library doesn't have the volume you seek, she may be able to suggest an alternative or direct you to the nearest library with the material you're looking for. The chief reference sources are:

1973 U.S. Physician Reference Listing (10 volumes). Clifton, N.J.: Fisher-Stevens, Inc., 1973.

This is a computerized printout of all physicians in the United States, giving their address, type of practice, specialty, board certification, specialty society, their year of birth, medical school, and year of graduation.

Directory of Medical Specialists. Chicago: A.N. Marquis Company, annual.

This lists those holding certification by the American Specialty Boards so that you can look up a particular type of specialist without having to know his name—just those who specialize, say, in your community or area.

American Dental Directory. Chicago: American Dental Association, annual.

Lists every dentist in the United States, giving his type of practice, whether on a dental school faculty, gives his date of birth, school from which graduated and when, address.

Cranin, A. Norman. *The Modern Family Guide to Dental Health.* New York: Stein and Day, 1971.

This is the first complete home dental reference book, a virtual encyclopedia of valuable information. Paperback edition also available.

AHA Guide to the Health Care Field.

This volume, published annually by the American Hospital Association (Chicago), tells you virtually everything you may want to know about a hospital—its size, services, affiliations, and whatever. Since it's sometimes put out under different titles you might have to ask your librarian.

There are other useful listings and compilations, but these vary with the community and state and year. Your librarian is usually up to date on what's going on, so ask.

Bibliography

American Medical Association, Committee on Human Sexuality. *Human Sexuality.* Chicago: American Medical Association, 1972.

Appraisal of Hospital Obsolescence. New York: Hospital Review and Planning Council of Southern New York, 1965.

Balint, M. *The Doctor, His Patient and the Illness.* Rev. ed. New York: International Universities Press, 1972.

Bird, B. *Talking with Patients.* 2nd ed. Philadelphia: J.B. Lippincott Company, 1973.

Brenton, Myron. *Sex Talk.* New York: Stein and Day, 1972.

Brodie, D.C. *Drug Utilization. . . .* Rockville, Md.: Department of Health, Education, and Welfare, 1970.

Bross, I.D.J., and Natarajan, N. "Leukemia from Low Level Radiation," *New England Journal of Medicine,* July 20, 1972.

Brown, J.A.C. *The Stein and Day International Medical Encyclopedia.* New York: Stein and Day, 1972.

Brown, R.F., *et al.* "Appraising Medical X-ray Protection Activities," *Practical Radiology,* April 1973.

Bunker, J.P. *The Anesthesiologist and the Surgeon.* Boston: Little, Brown and Company, 1972.

Cranin, A. Norman. *The Modern Family Guide to Dental Health.* New York: Stein and Day, 1971.

Denenberg, Herbert S. Lectures and pamphlet series, "A Shopper's Guide to. . . ." Harrisburg, Pa.: Pennsylvania Insurance Department.

"Eleventh Report of Human Renal Transplant Registry," *Journal of the American Medical Association,* December 3, 1973.

Frank, J.D. *Persuasion and Healing.* Baltimore: The Johns Hopkins Press, 1973.

Freeman, H.E., *et al. Handbook of Medical Sociology.* 2nd ed. Englewood Cliffs, N.J.: Prentice-Hall and Company, 1972.

Freidson, E. *Profession of Medicine.* New York: Dodd, Mead and Company, 1970.

Graham, J.B., and Paloucek, F.P. "Where Should Cancer of the Cervix Be Treated?" *American Journal of Obstetrics and Gynecology,* October 1, 1963.

Handbook of Non-Prescription Drugs. 1973 ed. Washington, D.C.: American Pharmaceutical Association, 1973.

"Hearings before Subcommittee on Monopoly," 92nd Congress, Parts 1, 2, and 3.

Kaulman, C. "There Ought to Be a Law Against X-ray Bunglers!" *Medical Economics,* October 23, 1972.

Kagan, B., and Fannin, S. "Spotlight on Antimicrobial Agents—1973," *Journal of the American Medical Association,* October 15, 1973.

Korsch, B.M., and Negrete, V.F. "Doctor-Patient Communication," *Scientific American,* August 1972.

Kunin, C.M., *et al.* "Use of Antibiotics," *Annals of Internal Medicine,* October 1973.

Lewis, C.E. "Variations in the Incidence of Surgery," *New England Journal of Medicine,* October 16, 1969.

Margulis, A.R. "The Lessons of Radiobiology . . . ," *American Journal of Roentgenology, Radium Therapy and Nuclear Medicine,* April 1973.

McClenahan, J.L. "Wasted X-rays," *Radiology,* August 1970.

Moses, L.E., and Mosteller, F. "Institutional Differences in Postoperative Death Rates," *Journal of the American Medical Association,* February 12, 1968.

"Reassessment of Surgical Specialty Training in the United States" (editorial), *Archives of Surgery,* June 1972.

"The Sick Physician," *Journal of the American Medical Association,* February 5, 1973.

Stewart, R.B., and Cluff, L.E. "Studies on the Epidemiology of Adverse Drug Reactions . . . ," *The Johns Hopkins Medical Journal,* December 1971.

Trussell, R. *The Quantity, Quality and Costs of Medical and Hospital Care Secured by a Sample of Teamster Families in the New York Area (1961).* New York: Columbia University School of Public Health and Administrative Medicine.

——. *A Study of the Quality of Health Care . . . (1964).*